LUNG CANCER

A PRACTICAL GUIDE TO MANAGEMENT

Fergus Macbeth
Western Infirmary,
Glasgow, Scotland

Robert Milroy
Stobhill Hospital,
Glasgow, Scotland

William Steward
Queen's University,
Kingston, Ontario, Canada

with

Rod Burnett
Western Infirmary, Glasgow, Scotland

harwood academic publishers
Australia • Canada • China • France • Germany • India
Japan • Luxembourg • Malaysia • The Netherlands • Russia
Singapore • Switzerland • Thailand • United Kingdom

Copyright © 1996 by OPA (Overseas Publishers Association) Amsterdam B.V. Published in The Netherlands by Harwood Academic Publishers GmbH.

Emmaplein 5
1075 AW Amsterdam
The Netherlands

British Library Cataloguing in Publication Data

Lung cancer: a practical guide to management
   1. Lungs – Cancer
   I. Macbeth, F.
   616. 9′9424

   ISBN 3-7186-5859-3 (Hardcover)
   ISBN 3-7186-5860-7 (Softcover)

CONTENTS

PREFACE

Lung cancer is a common problem and a major cause of morbidity and death. The generally poor prognosis of patients seems to have generated a degree of pessimism and lack of interest among the medical community. Lung cancer is more common than breast cancer, but if one compares them in terms of the resources devoted to the care of patients and to research, or of the number of specialist clinics and specialist surgeons and oncologists with a declared interest, lung cancer always seems to come a poor second.

This book has been written in an attempt to improve the overall understanding of lung cancer and the care of patients who suffer from it. This is deliberately not an exhaustive, heavily referenced academic tome, but rather, as the title states, a practical guide. We have tried to highlight important areas of controversy and debate, without going into too much detail, but have then given our own opinion of what the current best management might be. Above all, we have tried to give straightforward advice about managing problems, based on our own clinical experience, and we hope that not too much of it is idiosyncratic or controversial.

A number of important questions about the best treatment for lung cancer remain unanswered, and we would like to put in a plea for wider participation in clinical research. Many of these questions could be resolved by well-conducted multicentre clinical trials, but at the moment only a minority of patients are included in studies. We realize that participation in trials increases the work involved but we believe that it also increases the standard of care as well as being essential for future development.

Fergus Macbeth
Robert Milroy
William Steward

ACKNOWLEDGEMENTS

We are very grateful to Rod Burnett for his lucid chapter on the pathology of lung cancer.

We would also like to acknowledge the help and advice we have had from many colleagues in writing this book, especially Alan Kirk for his invaluable comments on surgical management and Mrs Betty McLean for her help with typing the manuscript. Finally, we would like to thank all the patients from whom we have, over the years, learnt so much.

1 EPIDEMIOLOGY AND AETIOLOGY

Lung cancer is a major cause of death in most Western countries and is an increasing health care problem in the developing nations. The World Health Organization estimates that nearly 6 million new patients are diagnosed with all forms of cancer each year and that two thirds of these will die. This represents 10% of all deaths and, in most countries, lung cancer is the most frequent cause of cancer deaths.

Although frustratingly few advances have been made in the treatment of lung cancer, a great deal is known about its aetiology. Despite the fact that the majority of cases could be prevented, its incidence continues to rise worldwide, and, as can be seen from Figure 1.1, the outcome for patients with lung cancer is dismal: only ten to fifteen percent survive one year from the time of diagnosis.

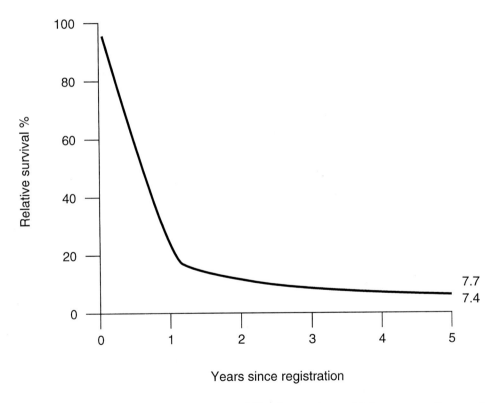

SURVIVAL - RELATIVE RATES

England & Wales 1981 Patients

Figure 1.1 Relative survival rates for United Kingdom patients with lung cancer diagnosed in 1981. (Reproduced with permission from Cancer Research Campaign 'Facts on Cancer'.)

INCIDENCE

Approximately 10% of all new patients diagnosed with cancer in the world have lung cancer. In 1980 there were estimated to be 660,500 new cases (513,600 males — 15.8% of cancers, 146,900 females — 4.7% of cancers) and the incidence is increasing by about 0.5% per year. There are approximately 161,000 new cases and 146,000 deaths per year in the United States and 45,000 new cases with 40,000 deaths per year in the United Kingdom.

The incidence of lung cancer varies widely between different countries. For men, Scotland has the highest national incidence in the world at 135/100,000 compared to 70/100,000 for the United States. The incidence is lower in Scandinavia at 44/100,000 and is only 7/100,000 in India. For women, the overall pattern is similar and the incidence is generally about a third of that in men. In recent years there has, however, been evidence in Western countries of a fall in the incidence of lung cancer in men with a continuing rise in the incidence in women. In Scotland, lung cancer has caused more deaths in women than breast cancer since 1988, and in Glasgow the incidence has been higher than that of breast cancer since 1990.

AETIOLOGY

Tobacco

A series of studies by Doll and colleagues,[1] using population groups of male British doctors, and by Hammond,[2] who investigated American men, established a link between the incidence of lung cancer and smoking. In the first study by Doll and Hill, which involved 40,637 British doctors, the risk of developing lung cancer in men who smoked more than 25 cigarettes a day was 25-fold greater than for non-smokers. This cohort was followed during a campaign to reduce cigarette consumption. The risk of developing lung cancer fell rapidly after stopping smoking and there was a 25% fall in lung cancer mortality over 12 years for male doctors compared with a 26% increase in a matched general population. Over the 12 years, the proportion of doctors who had stopped smoking increased from 20% to 32% and those who smoked cigarettes decreased from 41% to 21%. No reduction in cigarette consumption occurred in the general male population over the same time period.

There have been over thirty retrospective and eight prospective studies which have clearly established a link between cigarette smoking and lung cancer. It is estimated that 85–90% of all lung cancers can be linked to active smoking. The use of cigarettes carries a significantly greater risk of developing lung cancer than either pipe or cigar smoking (Table 1.1) and the risk is increased for those who inhale the smoke, take more inhalations from each cigarette, retain the cigarette in the mouth between inhalations and relight half-smoked cigarettes. It is possible that the reduced carcinogenic effect of pipe and cigar smoking is because less smoke is inhaled or because there is greater combustion of potential carcinogens.

Table 1.1 Lung cancer risks for pipe, cigar and cigarette smoking

Type of Smoking	Mortality Ratio
Never smoked regularly	1.00
Pipe and cigar	1.25
Cigar only	2.15
Pipe only	2.23
Cigarette and other	8.23
Cigarette only	10.08

The age of starting cigarette smoking, the duration of smoking and the nicotine content of the cigarettes are all important factors. The risk of lung cancer at the age of 60 years is three times greater for those who started smoking between the ages of 14 and 16 years compared to those who started 10 years later. It has been estimated that someone aged 35 years who smokes 25 or more cigarettes per day has a 13% chance of dying from lung cancer before the age of 75 years.

There has been a decline in smoking in both the United States and the United Kingdom. Between 1976 and 1987 the percentage of adult American men who smoked fell from 42% to 31%, and in women from 32% to 27%. The percentage decrease in the United Kingdom over the same time period was greater (falling from 49% of men in 1976 to 37% in 1986 and from 45% to 35 % of women). Of concern, however, is the fact that the group at most risk of developing lung cancer — those who begin smoking at an earlier age — has not decreased nearly as much as the overall population of smokers. In England and Wales approximately 18% of boys and 27% of girls between the ages of 15 and 16 years are regular smokers. A further disturbing feature is that in the United States, the percentage of men and women smoking more than 25 cigarettes a day has increased by 2% over the past 15 years. So although, in many countries the incidence of lung cancer appears to be declining in men and to be reaching a plateau in women, the disturbing trend of populations smoking greater numbers of cigarettes and starting at an earlier age may lead to a rise in incidence in future decades.

Despite the fall in cigarette consumption that has occurred over the past 20 years in Western Europe and the United States, tobacco production has actually increased (from about 600,000 to 700,000 tons per year in the United States between 1985 and 1994). As the domestic markets of the major international tobacco companies have shrunk, new markets have opened up to absorb this production, mainly in Asia, Africa and South America. Cigarettes are being promoted there with aggressive marketing targeted at groups who previously did not smoke, especially the young and women. As a result, tobacco consumption is actually rising worldwide. An example of this can be seen in Japan where the prevalence of smoking in women aged 20 to 29 years has increased by 50% in the past 18 years. If nothing is done to reduce this rising trend in cigarette smoking, the worldwide incidence of lung cancer will increase dramatically in the next 20 to 30 years. It has been estimated that as many as 2 or 3 million people may die every year by the year 2025.

It is important to be able to encourage smokers to stop their habit by telling them that the risk of developing lung cancer falls rapidly after they stop and that after 15 or 20 years as a non-smoker their risk will drop to only about twice that of life-time non-smokers.

Occupation and Lung Cancer Risk

Exposure to known carcinogens including asbestos, radon, chromium, nickel and inorganic arsenic compounds increases the risk of lung cancer. The association with occupational exposure to some of these agents seems to be independent of cigarette smoking, though, for asbestos, there may be a synergistic effect. Workers exposed to polycyclic aromatic hydrocarbons in chloromethyl ether are also at increased risk of developing lung cancer, particularly the small cell variant. It appears that there is a lag period of 10 to 25 years between exposure and developing overt cancer.

Asbestos

Asbestos exposure (particularly to the crocidolite or blue type) significantly increases the risk of developing lung cancer as well as malignant mesothelioma (see Chapter 14). This is seen in shipyard workers and in those who have been employed in the insulation, building, cement mixing and boiler-making industries. Even a short exposure may be sufficient to cause lung cancer, if the concentration of asbestos is high enough. There appears to be a synergistic effect of asbestos exposure and cigarette smoking, but it has recently been clearly demonstrated that non-smokers exposed to asbestos have a significantly higher risk of developing lung cancer varying between 1.5- and 30-fold higher than those not exposed. It has been estimated that in the West of Scotland, where there has been a large amount of industrial exposure to asbestos, about 6% of all lung cancers in men may be related directly to asbestos.[3]

Radon

Radon, a product of the decay of uranium-238, emits alpha particles and is found in some rocks, especially granites, and soils. It is an inert gas and can accumulate in buildings and mineshafts if ventilation is inadequate. There is no doubt that miners who are exposed to high concentrations of radon have an increased risk of lung cancer, but its role in domestic housing as a factor causing lung cancer is uncertain.

Diet

Some dietary factors have been implicated in causing lung cancer. Several agents including selenium, vitamins C and E and beta carotene have all been shown to scavenge free radicals, thus theoretically reducing some of the carcinogens produced by cigarette smoking and other pollutants. There is, however, no strong evidence that dietary deficiencies of these chemicals increase the risk of lung cancer. It has also been suggested that a high-fat diet may be a cofactor in the carcinogenesis of lung cancer.

Genetic Factors

The contribution of genetic factors to the development of lung cancer is being actively investigated. Several studies have shown an increased risk in the siblings of patients who develop lung cancer. Given the observation that almost all lung cancers are related to cigarette smoking, but only a relatively small percentage (10–15%) of smokers will develop lung cancer, several investigations have examined the potential of genetically inherited variations in the metabolism of carcinogens to affect risk.

The correlation between smokers' ability to metabolise the anti-hypertensive drug debrisoquine and their risk of developing lung cancer has been established. Metabolism of debrisoquine occurs through the cytochrome P-450 system and there is evidence that P-450 enzymes are also able to activate a chemical carcinogen in tobacco smoke. The activity of P-450 is inherited in a recessive manner and those who are fast metabolizers of debrisoquine have a significantly higher risk (approximately 8-fold) of developing lung cancer than those who are slow metabolizers.

Another candidate gene which may be associated with the risk of developing lung cancer is that encoding for glutathione-S-transferases. These proteins appear to be responsible for detoxifying polycyclic aromatic hydrocarbons and low levels may increase the risk of developing lung cancer caused by smoking. Other studies have linked deficiencies in enzymes responsible for repair of DNA-damage with increasing risks of developing lung cancer. Of particular interest is the inherited reduction or absence of the enzyme O^6-methylguanine-DNA methyl transferase.

Molecular genetic techniques can now be used to identify individuals with abnormal levels of enzyme expression. This gives the exciting prospect of being able to identify those at particular risk of developing lung cancer.

Chromosomal Abnormalities, Oncogenes and Growth Factors

An area of research that has expanded enormously in the past decade has been the investigation of genetic abnormalities which may be responsible for the development of lung cancer. Deletions of chromosomal material in the region 3p21 are seen in many lung cancers. The p53 gene may be mutated and altered expression of the p53 gene has been identified in some small and non-small cell lung cancers.

Altered expression of other oncogenes has also been demonstrated with different frequencies in the two main sub groups: cERB B2 and cFES are most frequently seen in non-small cell lung cancer (NSCLC) whereas nMYC appears to be specific for small cell lung cancer (SCLC). It is possible that these oncogenes have an effect by producing different growth factors or receptors and affecting critical areas of control of the cell cycle. An example is the production of the epidermal growth factor receptor by cERB B2. The addition of monoclonal antibodies to this receptor blocks the effect of epidermal growth factor and inhibits the growth of NSCLC cell lines *in vitro*.

With increasing understanding of the molecular events associated with the initiation, development and growth of lung cancers it may be possible to individualize treatments for different groups of patients. When, for example, specific growth factors or receptors are known to be up-regulated, the use of monoclonal antibodies specific for those factors may block their effects and slow or stop the rate of progression of the tumour. Protein kinases are activated following growth factor-receptor interactions and several inhibitors of these enzymes are being developed. The expression of particular oncogene products in resected specimens of NSCLC may be associated with a particularly poor prognosis, and patients who have undergone surgery and are found to have such abnormalities could, perhaps, be targeted for more intensive treatment. It seems likely that the understanding of the biology of lung cancer could soon provide more effective ways of preventing and treating this disease, but at the moment all these developments are experimental or theoretical and they have not yet reached routine clinical use.

KEY POINTS

- Lung cancer is the commonest cause of cancer deaths worldwide.
- Cigarette smoking causes 85–95% of cases of lung cancer.
- Although the incidence of lung cancer is declining in most developed countries, it is becoming an increasing problem in developing countries as cigarette smoking increases.
- Asbestos exposure appears to increase the risk of lung cancer.
- There may be some genetic factors, but their overall importance in the aetiology of lung cancer is not yet clear.

REFERENCES

1. Doll R., Peto R. (1976) Mortality in relation to smoking: 20 years' observation on male British doctors. *Br. Med. J.* **2,** 1525–1536.
2. Hammond E.C., Horn D. (1958) Smoking and death rates: report on 44 months of follow-up of 187,783 men. *J. Am. Med. Assoc.* **166,** 1294–1308.
3. Irvine H.D.V., Lamont D.W., Hole D.J., Gillis C.R. (1993) Asbestos and lung cancer in Glasgow and the West of Scotland. *Br. Med. J.* **306,** 1503–1506.

FURTHER READING

Charlton A. (1994) Tobacco and lung cancer. In *New Perspectives in Lung Cancer.* Edited by Thatcher N., Spiro S. pp. 1–18. London: BMJ Publishing Group.

2 CLINICAL PRESENTATION

The early detection of lung cancer gives the best chance of cure and so the possibility of an underlying tumour should always be considered in patients with risk factors who develop new or worsening respiratory symptoms. In particular this means middle-aged or elderly patients who are current or ex-smokers.

In this chapter we will describe the most frequent presenting symptoms, both respiratory and non-respiratory, and then discuss some of the more difficult clinical presentations in General Practice. Finally we will discuss how, when and where to refer for specialist advice.

CHEST SYMPTOMS

Cough and Sputum Production

Most patients with lung cancer have been or continue to be cigarette smokers and so cough and sputum production are common symptoms, but *increasing* cough and sputum production are sinister symptoms. An endo-bronchial tumour can directly stimulate sensory receptors in the airways and produce reflex coughing, or cause sputum retention due to impaired drainage. In addition, some lung tumours (especially broncho-alveolar carcinomas) are associated with increased mucus secretion and sputum production.

One of the most common presentations in General Practice is that of a middle-aged smoker with a recurrent or persistent chest infection. Patients at risk who have these symptoms for more than 3 weeks despite appropriate treatment must have a chest X-ray.

A 72-year-old, fit, male ex-smoker had minor symptoms of chronic bronchitis but during the preceding winter months he had three troublesome chest infections with increased cough and sputum production and a slight increase in breathlessness. These symptoms never fully resolved despite three courses of antibiotics. Physical examination was unremarkable but a chest X-ray showed a tumour in the right mid zone with right hilar enlargement. At bronchoscopy a non-small cell lung cancer was found in the right intermediate bronchus.

Breathlessness

Smokers are often breathless on exertion because of smoking-related chronic bronchitis and airflow obstruction, but *increasing* breathlessness is the second most common presenting symptom of lung cancer. This usually results from a proximal tumour partially or completely blocking a bronchus impairing airflow and drainage and causing collapse or consolidation of the distal lung.

The development of a significant pleural effusion is another common cause of breathlessness. Decreased lung compliance can occur with pulmonary metastases which will also result in breathlessness.

Wheeze

This is less frequently reported as a new symptom in patients with lung cancer. When it occurs, it is usually localised, does not change with coughing and does not respond to bronchodilator therapy.

Stridor is noisy inspiratory breathing due to upper airways narrowing and usually indicates major obstruction of the trachea or a main bronchus.

Haemoptysis

Haemoptysis is an alarming symptom and usually results in an early presentation for medical advice. Frequently it is only minor with some streaking in the sputum due to bleeding from the surface of the tumour, but occasionally it may be more substantial which suggests invasion of a blood vessel by the tumour. Only rarely is haemoptysis large enough to require urgent admission.

A smoker who has a single episode of even minor haemoptysis should have a chest X-ray and be referred to a Respiratory Physician for consideration of bronchoscopy.

> A 51-year-old male smoker presented with a single episode of haemoptysis. He was usually a little breathless on exertion and this had not got worse. Nothing abnormal was found on physical examination, but his chest X-ray showed a mass at the left hilum. Bronchoscopy demonstrated a squamous cell carcinoma in the left main stem bronchus.

Chest Pain

Non-specific vague chest discomfort can occur as the presenting symptom of lung cancer. It is often described as 'an ache inside the chest' or 'like toothache' and may be quite variable. More severe localised chest pain can occur and usually means tumour involvement of the mediastinum or parietal pleura, when it often has a more pleuritic character. Rib or intercostal nerve involvement can cause specific local chest pain often radiating round the chest wall in the course of the intercostal nerve.

Apical (Pancoast) tumours often present as shoulder ache and the misdiagnosis of a 'frozen shoulder' can result in weeks or months of delay before the correct diagnosis is made.

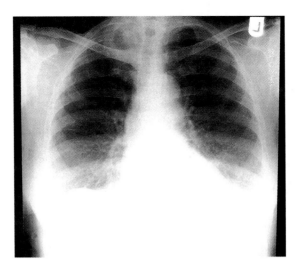

Plate 2.1   Chest X-ray of a patient presenting with right shoulder and chest wall pain, showing the classic features of a right sided Pancoast tumour, with erosion of the 3rd rib posteriorly.

> A 63-year-old man presented with a three-month history of right shoulder discomfort. His shoulder examination and X-ray were unremarkable, but over the next two months he developed weakness and sensory impairment in his right hand and the shoulder pain became more troublesome. A chest X-ray showed a right Pancoast tumour with rib erosion (Plate 2.1).

Symptoms of Local Tumour Extension

The primary tumour or mediastinal lymph node metastases may extend locally in the chest to involve any of the adjacent structures. A common problem is facial and upper limb swelling due to obstruction of the superior vena cava (See Chapter 11).

Direct infiltration of the oesophagus can result in dysphagia, and occasionally cause a tracheo- or broncho-oesophageal fistula with symptoms of paroxysmal cough on drinking or eating.

Local extension of the tumour may involve the left recurrent laryngeal nerve in its mediastinal course, causing vocal cord palsy and hoarseness, a common presenting symptom. Tumour infiltration of the cervical sympathetic chain in the root of the neck can result in Horner's syndrome (ipsilateral enophthalmos, miosis and lack of sweating on one side of the face), and direct extension into the brachial plexus (usually from an upper lobe tumour) can cause weakness and pain in the affected arm.

Infiltration of the pericardium can result in symptomatic cardiac arrhythmias, pericardial effusion (and occasionally tamponade) and pericarditic pain. Very occasionally the myocardium itself can be involved.

Extension of the tumour to the pleura may stimulate the production of pleural fluid and cause the symptoms associated with an effusion. Involvement of the chest wall itself may produce pain or even a local mass.

Symptoms of Widespread Metastases

Lung cancer often metastasises and the presenting symptoms may relate to extra-thoracic metastases. The common sites for symptomatic metastases are bone, liver and brain in decreasing order of frequency, but any organ can be involved.

Bone metastases usually present with pain and the commonest sites of symptomatic bony metastases are the spine, pelvis (especially sacro-iliac joints and around the hip), ribs and long bones. There is also a risk of pathological fracture especially of long bones.

Liver metastases are often asymptomatic but may cause anorexia and nausea, right upper quadrant discomfort from capsular distension or jaundice.

Brain metastases usually present with seizures, with progressive focal signs or, less commonly, with symptoms of raised intracranial pressure. Epilepsy occurring for the first time in a middle-aged smoker should raise suspicions of a metastasis and needs further investigation. Other neurological symptoms include cerebellar ataxia, hemiparesis, or more rarely personality change and confusion.

A 49-year-old, fit, male smoker with a slight cough presented with a single focal seizure. There were no residual neurological signs. He was referred for a chest X-ray which showed a small opacity lying behind the heart. Bronchoscopy demonstrated a small cell lung tumour in the posterior basal segment of the left lower lobe, and a CT scan of the brain confirmed cerebral metastases (Plate 2.2).

Lymph node and skin metastases can sometimes be the presenting problem. Lymph node metastases can occur almost anywhere and cause a variety of symptoms but the commonest sites are the supraclavicular fossae (especially the right side because of the drainage pattern). Isolated involvement of the lower cervical lymph nodes can occur with lung cancer but upper cervical lymphadenopathy suggests a primary head and neck tumour. Axillary node involvement is less common.

The intra-abdominal nodes may be involved and para-aortic lymphadenopathy occurs especially with lower lobe tumours. Enlarged para-aortic nodes may cause abdominal pain or obstruction of the duodenum or gastric outlet and enlarged nodes at the porta hepatis may cause jaundice.

Skin metastases noticed by the patient can be the presenting symptom. They are usually painless, purplish nodules, most commonly occurring on the trunk and, if left untreated may fungate and become infected.

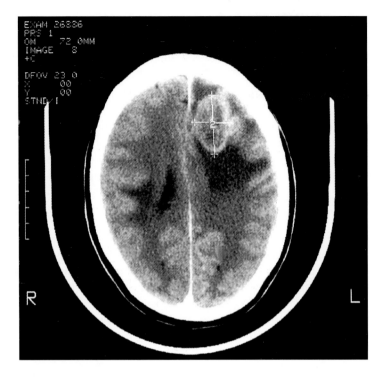

Plate 2.2   CT scan of brain showing a large metastatic deposit in the left frontal area. Note the surrounding oedema and midline shift.

Adrenal metastases are not uncommon but are usually asymptomatic. They may occasionally produce flank pain or haematuria from direct renal invasion, but adrenal failure and the symptoms of Addison's disease are most unusual.

Facial Pain

There is an unusual but well-recognised syndrome of facial pain in association with lung cancer, which may be the sole presenting symptom. It is characteristically a constant aching pain around the ear and angle of the jaw, though it may radiate

A 63-year-old smoker had left-sided facial pain for several months. Extensive investigation had revealed no obvious local cause. Treatment with simple analgesics, tricyclic antidepressants and carbamazepine had not controlled the pain and he was on increasing doses of morphine. A chest X-ray, after a single episode of haemptysis, revealed a mass at the left hilum, shown at bronchoscopy to be a large cell carcinoma. After a short course of palliative radiotherapy the facial pain improved and he was able to stop taking morphine.

further around the face, and on the same side as the tumour in the chest. It has been suggested that it may be caused by referred pain through the vagus nerve.

Patients with an otherwise unexplained or 'atypical' facial pain should have a chest X-ray to exclude lung cancer.

NON-METASTATIC EXTRA PULMONARY MANIFESTATIONS

A variety of para-neoplastic syndromes have been described and can be the cause of presenting symptoms.

Weight Loss

Weight loss is the commonest para-neoplastic symptom and is one which often worries patients greatly. In the absence of liver metastases or obstructive dysphagia it is probably related to the presence of circulating cytokines such as cachexin (tumour necrosis factor). It occurs in more than half of patients with lung cancer and indicates a relatively poor prognosis.

Finger Clubbing

Although finger clubbing occurs in a significant proportion of patients with lung cancer, it is rarely the presenting symptom of the disease (Plate 2.3).

Hypertrophic Pulmonary Osteoarthropathy (HPOA)

Joint pain and swelling caused by HPOA can occasionally be the presenting symptom of lung cancer. The pain typically occurs at the wrists and ankles but other large joints may be affected. The joints are often swollen and may be tender and finger clubbing (usually gross) is invariably present. The radiological changes are characteristic and consist of a calcifying periostitis near the joint and are best seen on X-rays of the wrist or ankle.

Endocrine Syndromes

These are discussed in detail in Chapter 9 and include:

Hypercalcemia
Hyponatremia due to inappropriate ADH secretion
Cushing's syndrome

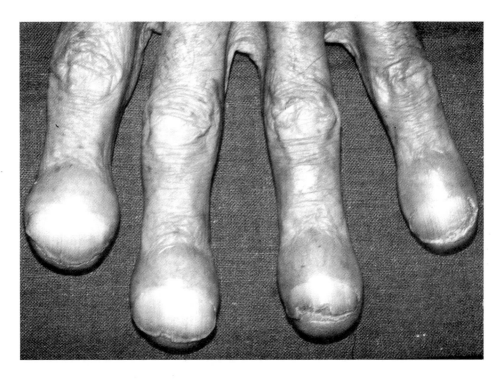

Plate 2.3   Gross finger clubbing in a patient with squamous cell lung carcinoma.

Non-metastatic Neurological Symptoms

These are discussed in detail in Chapter 10 and include:

> Cerebellar degeneration
> Peripheral neuropathy
> Spastic paraparesis
> Myopathy and myasthenia

Skin Problems

A number of unusual skin problems have been described in association with lung cancer including dermatomyositis, tylosis palmaris, acanthosis nigricans and hypertrichosis. Excess pigmentation secondary to ectopic ACTH is occasionally seen.

Coagulopathy

Lung cancer can be associated with various disorders of coagulation ranging from subtle disorders of haemostasis to overt thrombo-phlebitis migrans and deep venous thrombosis.

SIGNS OF LUNG CANCER

The clinical signs of lung cancer are as varied as the symptoms outlined above. They may be conveniently divided into local, metastatic and para-neoplastic. It should be emphasised, however, that if the history raises the possibility of lung cancer then a chest X-ray should be arranged even if there are no abnormal physical signs.

Local Signs

The earliest clinical signs of lung cancer are dullness to percussion and reduced breath sounds and vocal resonance on the side of the tumour. Other signs include those of lobar or pulmonary collapse, consolidation and pleural effusion. Invasion of the chest wall may be palpable.

The signs of early superior vena caval obstruction may sometimes be difficult to elicit. Always examine the neck veins carefully to see if there is any fullness or engorgement and also look at the chest wall for dilated superficial veins (Plate 2.4) and the face for peri-orbital oedema.

Signs of Distant Metastatic Disease

Because metastases from lung cancer can affect any part of the body, the possible clinical signs are many and varied. It is therefore important to carry out a thorough general physical examination, particularly if there are any suggestive symptoms.

Paraneoplastic Signs

About 25% of patients who present with lung cancer have finger clubbing. Gross finger clubbing is obvious (Plate 2.3) but the signs of early clubbing, oedema and loss of angle of the nail bed are more subtle and sometimes difficult to discern. Its cause remains obscure.

There may be evidence of weight loss or anaemia. Occasionally signs of para-neoplastic neurological syndromes, in particular cerebellar signs, may be present. Very rarely a patient may appear Cushingoid due to ectopic ACTH production.

PHYSICAL EXAMINATION

In order to manage the patient properly, it is crucial to know whether metastatic disease is present or not. It is therefore important always to examine for chest wall or spinal tenderness, examine the neck (from behind) for supra-clavicular and low cervical lymphadenopathy and the abdomen for an enlarged or tender liver. The absence of palpable hepatomegaly or liver tenderness does not however exclude micro-metastases in the liver. If there are any symptoms that suggest intracranial metastases then a careful neurological examination should be carried out and the

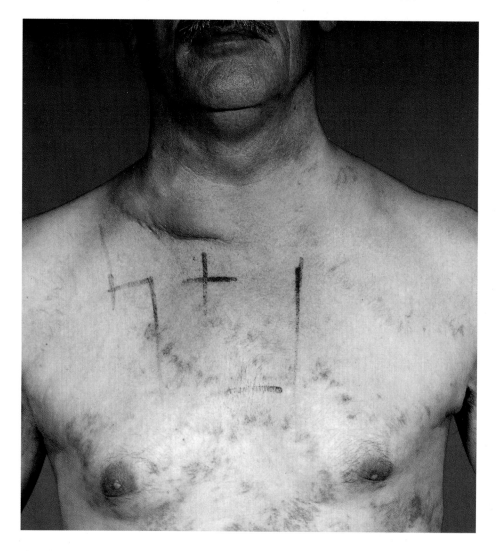

Plate 2.4 A patient with SVC obstruction with dilated neck veins and obvious collateral veins over the chest wall. The radiotherapy treatment field is marked.

signs of raised intracranial pressure (papilloedema, bradycardia and hypertension) sought.

HOW, WHEN AND WHERE TO REFER

In this chapter we have described the wide variety of ways in which patients with lung cancer can present. It is important always to be aware of the possibility that a smoker may have developed lung cancer, particularly because the only hope of cure is early diagnosis.

Any patient with symptoms suggesting lung cancer must have a chest X-ray. If this is suggestive of an intrathoracic tumour, the patient should be referred for specialist assessment by a Respiratory Physician. A smoker with haemoptysis should be referred even if the chest X-ray is normal. Depending on local practice either an urgent referral letter or a phone call should ensure that the patient is seen within a week.

The patient is examined to assess their general fitness, the presence or absence of metastatic disease, other medical conditions and lung function, and then further investigations will be arranged. Usually the patient will be bronchoscoped within a week of being seen and a treatment plan arranged within a fortnight of the patient being referred.

Clearly the pace of referral and investigations will depend on the patient's age and general fitness, because these will in part determine the eventual treatment options. Frail elderly patients should not be investigated vigorously because it unlikely that they will be subjected to intensive treatment.

The initial management of patients with symptoms suggestive of lung cancer is summarized in Figure 2.1.

KEY POINTS

- A smoker or ex-smoker with new respiratory symptoms which do not resolve within three weeks with antibiotic treatment should have a chest X-ray.
- A smoker or ex-smoker with haemoptysis should be referred for a specialist opinion even if the chest X-ray is normal.
- Shoulder pain radiating to the arm, facial swelling and facial pain can all be presenting symptoms of lung cancer.
- It is important to examine patients with suspected lung cancer for lymphadenopathy, chest wall or spinal tenderness and hepatomegaly.

FURTHER READING

Munro J., Edwards C. (1990) *McLeod's Clinical Examination*. Edinburgh: Churchill Livingstone,
Ogilvie C.M. (1990) Clinical Features. In *Respiratory Medicine*. Edited by Brewis R.A.L., Gibson G., Geddes D.M. pp. 207–221. London: Baillere Tindall.

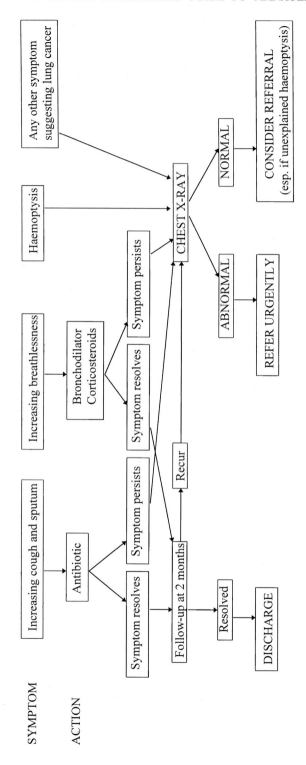

Figure 2.1   Managing the patient with symptoms suggestive of lung cancer.

3 INVESTIGATION

In this chapter we will describe the appropriate investigations for establishing the diagnosis of lung cancer and for defining the stage of disease.

RADIOLOGICAL INVESTIGATION OF THE CHEST

Chest X-Ray

A chest X-ray is the first investigation in someone suspected of having lung cancer. A single chest X-ray does not make the diagnosis but will often strongly suggest it and direct the relevant investigations.

In patients with a suspicious abnormality and no sputum production, but who have very poor lung function and are unsuitable for bronchoscopy, a repeat chest X-ray after an interval of around three months may show the lesion to have grown and thus confirm the presence of a tumour.

A lateral film can be useful in localizing abnormalities seen on a postero-anterior (PA) chest X-ray or in showing up a tumour behind the heart that is not otherwise visible.

A normal chest X-ray does not exclude the diagnosis of lung cancer, and a smoker with haemoptysis should be investigated further even if the chest X-ray is normal.

By the time a patient's lung cancer is causing symptoms, the chest X-ray is usually abnormal. A wide variety of abnormalities may be seen (see Plates 2.1, 3.1, 3.2, 3.3) including:

- peripheral, hilar or paratracheal mass lesions
- collapse or consolidation of a lobe or whole lung
- pleural thickening or effusion
- elevated hemidiaphragm
- apical opacity (Pancoast tumour)
- pulmonary metastases
- rib erosion
- bone metastases

The chest X-ray should be carefully examined and a number of specific underlying abnormalities looked for:

- The volumes of both lungs should be studied as loss of volume on one side, indicated by mediastinal shift and changes in the position of the hemidiaphragm, implies partial collapse and the possibility of an underlying tumour.
- The lung apices must be examined carefully for the opacification and rib erosion seen in a Pancoast tumour (see Plate 2.1).

19

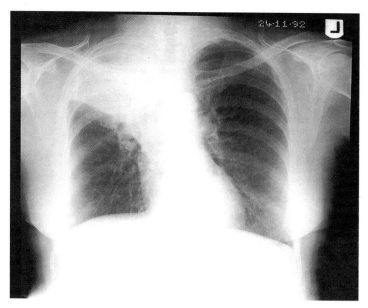

Plate 3.1   Chest X-ray showing collapse of the right upper lobe from a squamous cell carcinoma occluding the right upper lobe bronchus.

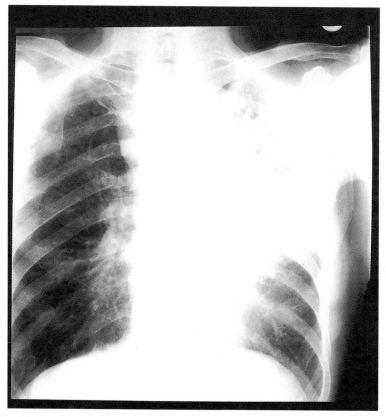

Plate 3.2   Chest X-ray of a patient with small cell lung cancer showing consolidation of the left upper lobe and right para-tracheal lymphadenopathy.

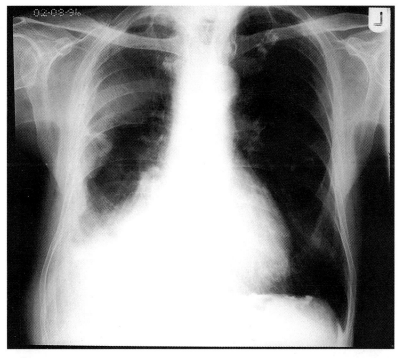

Plate 3.3 Chest X-ray showing extensive left-sided pleural calcification, loss of volume of the right lung and a lobulated pleural mass, typical of a mesothelioma.

- If a mass is visible, erosion of adjacent ribs should be looked for, especially if the patient has chest wall pain and tenderness.
- Mediastinal widening suggesting mediastinal lymphadenopathy (and inoperability) can also be missed if not specifically looked for.

Computerised Tomographic (CT) Scanning

CT scanning is not needed for many patients with lung cancer but is essential for the assessment before surgery or radical radiotherapy and is important in the evaluation of mesothelioma. See Plates 3.4, 3.5.

Modern CT scanners, with short scanning times and less movement artefact, usually give good images of the primary tumour, but it is sometimes difficult to distinguish tumour tissue from distal consolidation. It is often possible to get an indication of whether there is invasion of mediastinal structures or the chest wall. Partial volume effects, however, may limit the accuracy of the assessment.

The following findings on CT scanning are very suggestive of mediastinal invasion and therefore of inoperability:

- compression of mediastinal vessels or oesophagus
- loss of the fat plane usually seen around mediastinal blood vessels
- tumour mass in contact with more than 25% of the aortic circumference
- tumour in contact with more than 3 cm of the mediastinum

Mediastinal lymph nodes can often be identified, but even if they are significantly enlarged, it does not necessarily mean that they are involved with tumour.

The upper abdomen can be scanned at the same time as the chest to exclude liver and adrenal metastases.

CT scanning can also be used to guide transthoracic, diagnostic fine needle biopsies.

Magnetic Resonance (MR) Scanning

Compared to CT, MR scanning has both advantages and disadvantages for anatomical staging. CT scanning is better for detecting and evaluating pulmonary nodules, parenchymal abnormalities and, probably, pleural abnormalities and fluid collections,

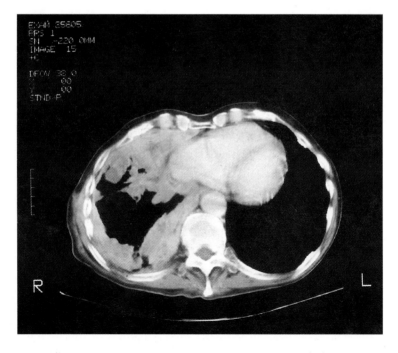

Plate 3.4 CT scan of the chest of the same patient as Plate 3.3, showing an extensive pleural-based tumour encircling the right lung and growing into the fissure, and also chest wall involvement.

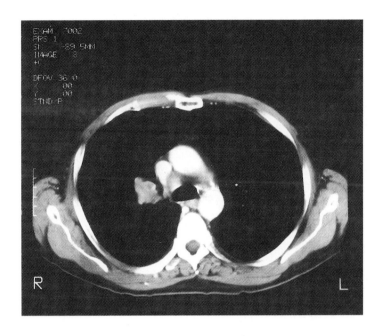

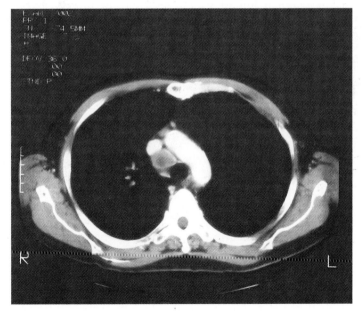

Plate 3.5 CT scan of the chest of a patient with tumour at the right hilum (upper) and mediastinal lymphadenopathy (lower).

because of its better spatial resolution and ability to detect calcification. CT scanning can also clearly image the bronchial abnormalities that are common in patients with lung cancer.

Because of its ability to discriminate between some tissues, MR scanning appears to be better than CT for assessing chest wall invasion, imaging Pancoast tumours and distinguishing between tumour and distal collapse and consolidation. This partly relates to volume-averaging problems that can occur on transaxial CT scans and are avoided or clarified by MR.

For the assessment of the hila and mediastinum, especially the extent of nodal involvement, CT and MR scanning provide similar information.

Although MR scanning has the advantage of no radiation and providing sagittal and coronal images, CT remains the routine investigation of choice for the intrathoracic staging of patients with lung cancer. It is more widely available, less expensive and its role is well established. MR may be preferable in the assessment of chest wall invasion and Pancoast tumours, and in patients whose CT scan findings are confusing or equivocal.

CONFIRMING THE DIAGNOSIS

To confirm the diagnosis of lung cancer, histopathological or cytological evidence of malignancy must be obtained. The precise histology has major implications for further investigation and treatment and for prognosis. There are three main ways of making a histological diagnosis: sputum cytology, sampling at bronchoscopy and biopsy of metastases.

Sputum Cytology

Cytological examination of the sputum is a useful and undervalued technique and, for frail patients, it offers the chance of making a diagnosis non-invasively.

The yield from sputum cytology increases as more samples are examined and at least three specimens should be sent to the laboratory. It is also important that mucoid secretions from the lower airways and not saliva are examined. Physiotherapy (sometimes with sputum induction using hypertonic saline) can be helpful in obtaining satisfactory specimens. Sputum obtained after bronchoscopy has a high diagnostic yield and this should be requested routinely in patients suspected of having lung cancer if no definite tumour was seen at bronchoscopy.

Bronchoscopy

The usual method of making a diagnosis of lung cancer is by bronchoscopy and biopsy, and bronchoscopy is essential in the work-up of patients being considered for surgery.

Although fibre-optic bronchoscopy can be done quite easily without significant upset for most patients, it is important to consider the patient's respiratory reserve beforehand. If there is any history to suggest poor respiratory function, spirometry and measurement of arterial oxygen tension must be carried out.

Bronchoscopy is usually done on an out-patient (daycase) basis (Plate 3.6) and takes about 20 minutes. Patients usually receive some form of intravenous sedation (e.g. diazepam or midazolam) and also often an anticholinergic drug (atropine 0.6 mg) to reduce bronchial secretions.

There are many techniques for applying topical anaesthesia. Benzocaine lozenges can be sucked before the procedure and are useful as a preliminary to the application of local anaesthetic. If a standard nasal approach is used, the nares are normally anaesthetized with topical lignocaine spray and jelly. The larynx is then anaesthetized with 2 ml aliquots of 4% lignocaine. Further aliquots are trickled through the larynx into the trachea, and then applied via the bronchoscope to the upper lobes. Some of

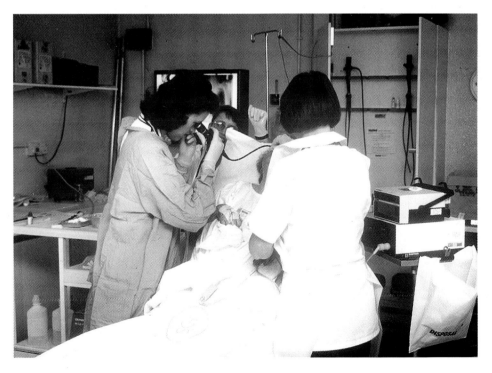

Plate 3.6 Fibreoptic bronchoscopy. The patient is lying comfortably and is being monitored (pulse oximeter and ECG).

the local anaesthetic will then pass down to the lower lobe bronchi. Alternatively, nebulized lignocaine can be inhaled or cocaine injected below the larynx via a transcricoid fine needle puncture.

Once satisfactory sedation and topical anaesthesia have been achieved, the lubricated bronchoscope can usually be passed through a nostril fairly easily.

If it is not possible to pass the bronchoscope through the nose because the nares are very narrow or there has been previous nasal trauma, the bronchoscope sometimes has to be passed through the mouth using an appropriate tooth-guard to prevent trauma to the bronchoscope.

At bronchoscopy, the oropharynx, larynx, trachea, carina and all lobar and segmental orifices can usually be clearly seen and carefully examined.

In patients being considered for surgical resection it is important to examine the vocal cords for evidence of palsy. This would suggest that the tumour has invaded the mediastinum and involved the recurrent laryngeal nerve, which would make the patient inoperable.

For similar reasons the trachea has to be examined carefully because tumour here excludes curative surgery and if the carina is splayed (indicating significant subcarinal lymphadenopathy) a curative surgical resection will not be possible (see Chapter 6).

At bronchoscopy, lung cancer may appear as an obvious polypoid tumour, sometimes with necrotic tumour on the surface, or simply as a sub-mucosal infiltrate. Biopsies can easily be taken under direct vision using forceps passed through the bronchoscope. Bleeding may occur but is not usually a significant problem. Even if tumour is not seen at bronchoscopy it is often possible to make a diagnosis of lung cancer by passing brushes into the affected area of lung and then washing with saline (20 ml aliquots).

The diagnostic yield from biopsies taken at bronchoscopy is high, but the diagnosis can also often be made from cytological examination of brush specimens and bronchial aspirate, as well as post-bronchoscopy sputum specimens.

The complication rate from fibre-optic bronchoscopy is small if patients are selected appropriately. Nowadays, patients have their pulse and oxygen saturation monitored during the procedure because transient hypoxemia and the effects of lignocaine can result in cardiac dysrhythmias and, occasionally, oversedation can result in transient respiratory failure. These complications can be avoided by careful selection of patients, sensible administration of drugs, using oxygen as appropriate, and monitoring the patient during the procedure.

Transbronchial and Percutaneous Biopsy

Sometimes it is not possible to make a diagnosis from bronchoscopy. If there is a mass lesion clearly visible on the chest X-ray, either transbronchial lung biopsy or percutaneous transthoracic needle aspiration can be used to obtain specimens.

Transbronchial lung biopsy is done at the time of bronchoscopy. The biopsy forceps are passed out to the lesion and biopsies can be taken under fluoroscopic control.

This procedure is only used if tumour is not accessible at a routine bronchoscopy because it carries a higher risk of haemorrhage and a small risk of pneumothorax.

Transthoracic, fine needle aspiration is carried out under fluoroscopic or CT scanning control. This procedure is relatively simple to perform but again carries a significant risk (about 15%) of causing a pneumothorax, although this is not usually large enough to require intercostal drainage.

Pleural Aspiration and Biopsy

In a patient with a significant pleural effusion shown on chest X-ray, a diagnosis may be made on cytology of the pleural fluid or on histology of a pleural biopsy. We recommend that a pleural aspiration is the first procedure, and, if this does not yield a diagnosis that this is repeated and followed by a pleural biopsy. Pleural biopsy is a more invasive procedure and is associated with a significant risk of bleeding and pneumothorax.

Pleural aspiration is a straightforward procedure. The site of aspiration can be determined by clinical examination, review of the chest X-ray, or, if there is only a small fluid collection, by ultrasound localisation.

- Sit the patient comfortably, bent forwards over the back of a chair.
- Clean the skin and infiltrate 2 to 4 ml of 2% lignocaine (without adrenaline) into the skin and then the intercostal muscles.
- Aim through the intercostal space, keeping just above the lower rib, to avoid the neuro-vascular bundle.
- Advance the needle cautiously, and suck back before injecting local anaesthetic, to ensure that a blood vessel has not been entered.
- Once the pleural space is entered, yellowish or blood-stained fluid will be aspirated.
- Allow a few minutes for the local anaesthetic to take effect.
- Insert the pleural aspiration needle, attached to a three way tap and syringe. A significant 'give' is usually felt when the pleural space is entered.
- Aspirate samples for cytology, bacteriology and biochemistry.

Pleural biopsy is carried out in a similar way to aspiration, but using a pleural biopsy needle (e.g. Abraham's needle). It is a potentially hazardous procedure and should only carried out after supervised instruction.
- Prepare the skin and anaesthetize the intercostal space as above.
- Make a small skin incision with a scalpel blade.
- Dissect bluntly down between the ribs with forceps.
- Gently insert the pleural biopsy needle in the 'closed' position until the pleural space is entered, open the needle and suck back pleural fluid.
- Withdraw the needle in the 'open' position until the aperture snares on the parietal pleura.
- Close the aperture to obtain the sample with a twising action and withdraw the needle.

- Repeat at least three times.
- Get a chest X-ray to ensure that a pneumothorax has not been produced.

Biopsy of Metastases

If there are obvious metastatic deposits that are easily biopsied, bronchoscopy may not be needed. In particular the supraclavicular fossae should be examined for nodes and the skin for deposits which can be excised or needled. Sometimes the diagnosis is made by biopsying liver, bone or, occasionally, brain metastases.

Fine needle aspiration is a quick and simple procedure.

- Identify the lesion to be aspirated and clean the overlying skin.
- Infiltrate the skin with a small amount of local anaesthetic (up to 1 ml of 2% lignocaine).
- Fix the lesion with one hand, which also applies tension to the skin surface.
- Pass a needle attached to a plastic syringe into the lesion, which often feels 'gritty' as the needle is passed through.
- Apply gentle suction to the syringe plunger and pass the needle up and down inside the lesion without taking the needle tip back out to the surface.
- Withdraw the needle and syringe gently and release the pressure just as the needle is pulled out of the lesion. The majority of the cells stay in the needle and air and blood are not sucked up into the syringe as the needle is removed.
- Expel the material in the needle and syringe onto a glass slide which can then be air-dried and stained for examination.

Table 3.1   Causes of abnormal biochemistry in patients with lung cancer

Abnormality	Causes
Raised alkaline phospatase	Bone metastases
	Liver metastases
	Obstructive liver disease
	Paget's disease
Hypercalcaemia	Bone metastases
	Ectopic PTH (squamous carcinoma)
Abnormal liver function tests	Liver metastases
	Alcoholic liver damage
	Other liver disease
Hyponatraemia	SIADH (small cell lung cancer)

SCREENING FOR METASTASES

When a diagnosis of lung cancer has been made, the question of how thoroughly to assess the extent of the disease has to be considered. In frail patients extensive screening investigations for metastatic disease are not necessary, but if a patient is being considered for surgical resection or radical radiotherapy, then he or she should be investigated carefully. In patients with small cell lung cancer, the presence of metastatic disease may determine the chemotherapy regimen.

History and Physical Examination

The presence of metastases may be suspected or confirmed by careful history and examination (see Chapter 2). Symptoms which should make one suspicious include anorexia, weight loss, hoarseness, bony pain and epigastric or right upper quadrant discomfort.

It is important to examine the patient specifically for supraclavicular and cervical lymphadenopathy, bone tenderness, hepatomegaly, Horner's syndrome and skin deposits.

Blood Tests

The essential blood investigations are a full blood count, and measurement of the serum calcium, alkaline phosphatase and liver function tests.

Abnormal biochemistry does not necessarily mean that there is metastatic disease and the various causes are listed in Table 3.1.

Liver Imaging

Imaging of the liver is indicated if there is palpable hepatomegaly or abnormal liver function tests. If there is no clinical evidence to suggest liver metastases then the diagnostic yield of routine screening is low. Even so, in patients being considered for surgery or radical radiotherapy it should still be done because the liver is the common site of asymptomatic metastases.

Liver ultrasound is the preferred technique for screening for liver metastases because, in most hospitals, it is the most sensitive, as well as being non-invasive and relatively cheap. A normal ultrasound of liver cannot, however, reliably exclude micro-metastases.

CT scanning of the liver is slightly less sensitive than ultrasound but may be convenient if the patient is having a chest CT anyway as part of the preoperative assessment.

Isotope scanning of the liver has been superseded by ultrasound and CT.

Isotope Bone Scanning

Bone scanning is indicated if there is clinical or biochemical evidence to suggest bone metastases. There may, however, be problems in interpreting bone scans: arthritis, osteoporosis in the spine with vertebral body collapse, previous trauma and Paget's disease can all cause difficulties.

It is therefore important to relate the bone scan abnormalities to the clinical story and current X-rays; very occasionally a bone biopsy may be necessary.

CT Scanning of the Brain

A CT scan of the brain is only necessary if the patient has symptoms or signs to suggest central nervous system (CNS) metastases (see Plate 2.2). It is not part of the routine staging of patients, although some centres include it in the preoperative assessment of patients with adenocarcinoma because of the relatively high incidence of brain metastases with this tumour type.

Isotope brain scanning is less sensitive and only has a role as a screening test when access to CT scanning is difficult. If an isotope brain scan is normal and CNS metastases are suspected clinically then a CT scan of brain must be performed.

ASSESSMENT OF LUNG FUNCTION

Assessment of lung function is only required for patients who are being considered for surgery or radical radiotherapy. A few simple questions in the history may give enough information. If a patient is breathless after walking for 50 yards on the flat or up a slight incline, then further tests are not needed as surgery or radical radiotherapy are clearly not feasible.

If the patient appears clinically to have satisfactory lung function then it is important to carry out formal tests including lung volumes, gas transfer and arterial blood gas analysis. However, if the patient is young, fit and has excellent exercise tolerance these investigations are unnecessary.

There are three categories of patients who can cause problems:

- Patients with adequate measured lung volumes who seem clinically to be limited. This may reflect impaired diffusion with desaturation on exercise and measurement of gas transfer is therefore an important part of lung function assessment.
- Patients with adequate lung function who cough and desaturate during bronchoscopy are usually less attractive candidates for surgery.
- Patients with borderline lung function tests who appear clinically to have satisfactory exercise tolerance. Assessing their exercise capacity (by either a formal walking test or simply asking them to walk round the hospital on the flat and up stairs) can help in deciding whether surgery or radical radiotherapy are feasible.

KEY POINTS

- The investigation of a patient suspected of having lung cancer is summarized   in Figure 3.1.
- A normal chest X-ray does not exclude the diagnosis of lung cancer.
- A lateral chest X-ray can be useful in localizing abnormalities seen on the PA chest X-ray.
- Fibre-optic bronchoscopy and biopsy are usually the best way to confirm the diagnosis.
- CT scanning of the chest and upper abdomen is an essential part of assessing patients for surgery and radical radiotherapy.
- CT scanning of the brain and isotope bone scanning are only necessary if metastases are suspected clinically.
- Formal lung function tests are useful in assessing patients for surgery, but it is important to consider the patient's actual exercise tolerance as well.

FURTHER READING

Muers M.F. (1994) How much investigation? In *New Perspectives in Lung Cancer.* Edited by Thatcher N., Spiro S. pp. 77–104. London: BMJ Publishing Group.

Hanson P., Collins J. (1990) Bronchoscopy and lavage. In *Respiratory Medicine.* Edited by Brewis R.A.L., Gibson G., Geddes D.M. pp. 316–329. London: Baillere Tindall.

Felson B. (1973) *Chest Roentgenology.* Philadelphia: W.B. Saunders.

Armstrong P., Wilson A.G., Dee P. (1990) Bronchial carcinoma and mesothelioma. In *Imaging Disease of the Chest.* pp. 258–349. St Louis: Mosby Year Book.

Haaga J., Lanzieri C.F., Sartoris D.J., Zerhouni E.A. (1994) Bronchial carcinoma. In *Computed Tomography and Magnetic Resonance Imaging of the Whole Body.* pp. 713–736. St Louis: Mosby Year Book.

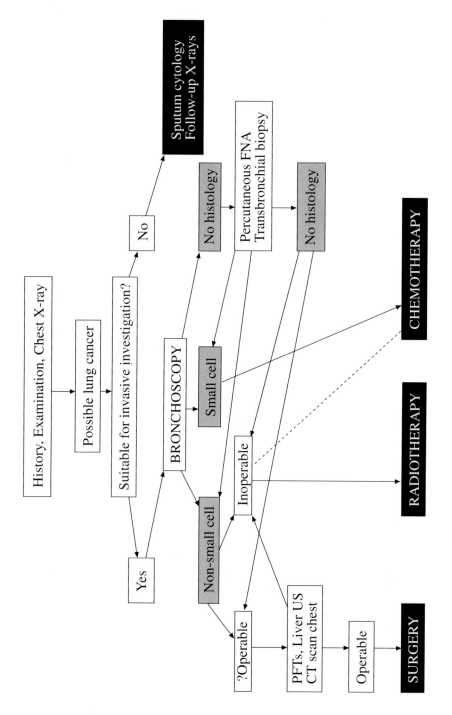

Figure 3.1   Investigation of the patient with possible lung cancer.

4 THE PATHOLOGY OF LUNG CANCER

INTRODUCTION

The histopathologist has a major role in the diagnosis and management of lung cancer. Because of the serious implications of such a diagnosis, it is important that a 'robust' pathological diagnosis is obtained, by either histopathological or cytological methods. Furthermore, once a diagnosis of cancer has been made, the histological type must be well characterized before appropriate therapy can be chosen. The pathologist may also be required when examining resection specimens or other biopsies (e.g. mediastinal biopsies) to give an opinion on the degree of spread of the tumour (i.e. staging).

A variety of techniques are used to obtain material for histological and cytopathological examination. The simplest of these is the examination of sputum for exfoliated malignant cells. Unfortunately, sputum is easily contaminated by saliva, oral squames and bacteria, and better cytological specimens are usually obtained during bronchoscopy by bronchial washing and bronchial brushing. The mainstay of histopathological diagnosis is a bronchial biopsy carried out during bronchoscopy, after a suspicious lesion has been detected. Transbronchial lung biopsy may sometimes be used to obtain material from lesions further out in the periphery of the lung. Pleural lesions and very peripheral tumours may be susceptible to diagnosis by percutaneous pleural and lung needle biopsy. Occasionally, when all these methods fail, an open approach may be necessary, and material may be removed at thoracotomy and submitted to a rapid diagnostic procedure (frozen section). Other techniques such as cervical lymph node biopsy or mediastinoscopy may obtain tumour tissue suitable for histological examination.

CLASSIFICATION

In 1967 the World Health Organization published the first widely accepted histological classification of lung cancer,[1] but this was subsequently modified considerably, and the most extensively used classification currently is the World Health Organization's second histological classification published in 1981[2] (Table 4.1) which will subsequently be referred to in this chapter as WHO2.

WHO2 subdivides the main types of lung cancer into four different categories:

1. Squamous cell carcinoma
2. Small cell carcinoma
3. Adenocarcinoma
4. Large cell carcinoma

The two main differences between the original World Health Organization classification and WHO2 are that in WHO2 the small cell carcinoma group was

Table 4.1   WHO-1981 Histological Classification of Lung Tumours.

A. BENIGN:
   1. Papillomas:
      (a) Squamous cell papilloma
      (b) 'Transitional' papilloma
   2. Adenomas:
      (a) Pleomorphic adenoma ('mixed' tumour)
      (b) Monomorphic adenoma
      (c) Others

B. DYSPLASIA
   CARCINOMA IN SITU

C. MALIGNANT:
   1. Squamous cell (epidermoid) carcinoma:
      Variant:
      (a) Spindle cell (squamous) carcinoma
   2. Small cell carcinoma:
      (a) Oat cell carcinoma
      (b) Intermediate cell type
      (c) Combined oat cell carcinoma
   3. Adenocarcinoma:
      (a) Acinar adenocarcinoma
      (b) Papillary adenocarcinoma
      (c) Broncho-alveolar carcinoma
      (d) Solid carcinoma with mucus formation
   4. Large cell carcinoma:
      Variants:
      (a) Giant cell carcinoma
      (b) Clear cell carcinoma
   5. Adenosquamous carcinoma
   6. Carcinoid tumour
   7. Bronchial gland carcinomas:
      (a) Adenoid cystic carcinoma
      (b) Mucoepidermoid carcinoma
      (c) Others
   8. Others

---

simplified and large cell tumours which produced mucin were included in the adenocarcinoma group rather than the large cell anaplastic group. These four carcinoma groups form the vast majority of all lung cancers and discussion and description of these will form the bulk of this chapter. Brief consideration will be given to the rarer types of lung cancer and to the relatively uncommon benign tumours.

Central and Peripheral Tumours

Between 70% and 80% of lung cancers arise centrally, that is from main or segmental bronchi. All four main histological types of lung cancer may arise in this way and all are regarded as being smoking-related cancers. Clearly these tumours can be diagnosed by endobronchial biopsy. About 20% of lung cancers arise from the lung parenchyma itself, and are apparently not associated with a major bronchus. In the remainder of cases the exact origin of the tumour cannot be determined. Many of the peripherally arising tumours do not appear to be related to smoking cigarettes.

It should be appreciated that when used pathologically, the terms 'centrally-arising' and 'peripherally-arising' apply to the origin of the tumour from a major airway and this may or may not correspond to the radiological use of the terms 'central' and 'peripheral' tumours.

HISTOLOGICAL TYPES

Squamous Cell Carcinoma

Squamous cell carcinoma (Plate 4.1a) is the commonest type of lung cancer seen in the United Kingdom. It usually arises centrally and is uncommon in non-smokers. Because of differences in the exact classification of lung cancer, it is not possible to give reliable figures as to the exact proportion of lung cancers that are squamous. In the WHO2 classification, squamous cell carcinomas may only be diagnosed if the carcinoma shows either keratin production or if the cells have clear intercellular bridges ('prickles').

Squamous cell carcinoma of the bronchus occurs following metaplasia of the pseudostratified, ciliated, bronchial epithelium into squamous epithelium and dysplastic squamous epithelium ('in situ carcinoma') may frequently be seen adjacent to invasive squamous cell carcinomas of the bronchus in resection specimens. Squamous carcinoma, particularly if well differentiated, offers the best prognosis of all of the four main types of lung cancer and is most amenable to surgical resection. It tends to grow relatively slowly and produces symptoms and signs in relation to the local 'mass' lesion such as haemoptysis or persistent chest infection due to bronchial obstruction. Squamous cell carcinoma tends to metastasise relatively late and even then initially to local lymph nodes.

Patients who have been successfully treated by surgical resection for squamous cell carcinoma of the bronchus sometimes return some five to ten years later with another squamous cell carcinoma of the contralateral lung. This is a reflection of the squamous metaplasia/dysplasia field change in the bronchial epithelium and most of these tumours are regarded as second primary carcinomas rather than recurrences. The use of agents such as vitamin A and beta-carotenes has been advocated in an attempt to reverse this dysplastic-field change and reduce the risk of a second primary carcinoma.

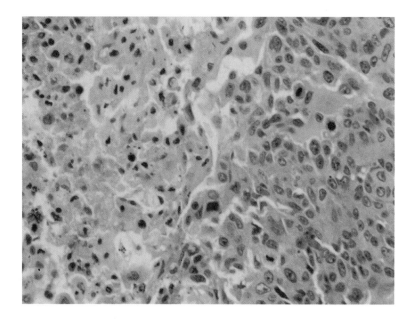

Plate 4.1a   Squamous carcinoma. This is composed of large pink tumour cells. There is extensive keratin production seen on the left-hand side of the photomicrograph.

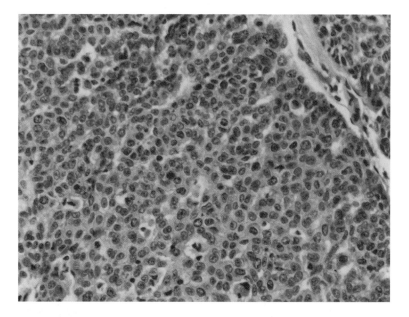

Plate 4.1b   Small cell carcinoma. The tumour cells are much smaller, closely packed and polygonal. In the classic 'oat cell' type the cells are even smaller and fusiform in shape.

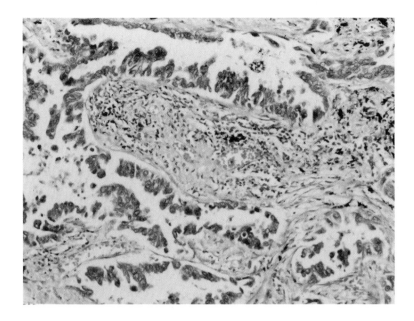

Plate 4.1c Adenocarcinoma. The tumour cells are forming glandular structures. Some of these tumours produce mucin.

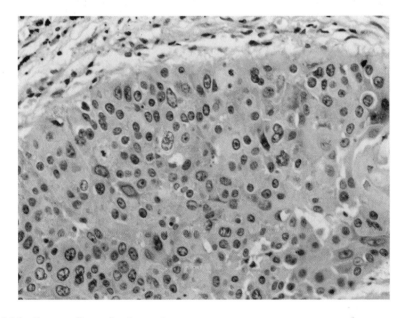

Plate 4.1d Large cell anaplastic carcinoma.

Small Cell Carcinoma ('Oat' Cell Carcinoma)

These are highly malignant neuroendocrine carcinomas which arise from cells of the diffuse neuroendocrine system (Plate 4.1b) that are normally present in the air passages (Feyrter cells). These tumours almost invariably arise centrally and are smoking-related. In contrast to the squamous cell carcinomas, they are rapidly spreading tumours and frequently present with metastases. The tumour cells may be relatively small and round with little cytoplasm (lymphocyte-like) or somewhat larger and fusiform (classical 'oat'cell type) or of relatively nondescript or 'polygonal' cell type. Apart from these true 'small' cell tumours, a variant known as the 'intermediate' cell type of small cell carcinoma consists of considerably larger cells, although it maintains the same histological characteristics as its smaller cell variants. This tumour type must not be confused with the large cell anaplastic group. Occasionally, small cell tumours are mixed with other types of lung cancer, particularly with squamous cell carcinoma and WHO2 regards these as combined oat cell carcinomas (category 2c). The question of heterogeneity in lung cancer is considered below.

Small cell carcinoma is the most malignant type of lung cancer and is capable of very rapid growth, although, paradoxically, the primary tumour itself may be relatively small. The hilar mass frequently seen with this type of tumour represents nodal involvement rather than the primary tumour itself, and, by this time small cell cancer is likely to be widely disseminated.

Adenocarcinoma

Adenocarcinoma of the lung (Plate 4.1c) is a complex group of tumours even if the bronchial gland tumours are excluded (see below). Centrally arising adenocarcinomas are the least common of the major groups, although they are also caused by smoking. They may be acinar or papillary in appearance and their degree of differentiation varies considerably. They tend to be more aggressive than squamous cell carcinoma, but do not spread as rapidly as the small cell type of tumour. Adenocarcinoma of the lung may also arise peripherally and two special types are recognized.

Bronchoalveolar carcinoma

Bronchoalveolar carcinoma is an adenocarcinoma which arises peripherally and may form a relatively large mass before it comes to diagnosis. Growth is of variable rapidity and the tumour may be multicentric or even bilateral. A recurrent pneumonic presentation is not unusual and occasionally these tumours may secrete large amounts of mucus which leads to the clinical symptom of bronchorrhea. They tend to spread throughout the lung parenchyma, without causing destruction, by growing along the alveolar walls (so-called lepidic spread). Because of their growth pattern these tumours may spread widely within the lung parenchyma and involve several lobes or even the contralateral lung, spread being by intrabronchial metastasis.

Scar Carcinoma

Some peripheral carcinomas of the lung, usually adenocarcinomas, appear to arise in old scars (Plate 4.2). There is considerable controversy about the frequency of this occurrence, although most authorities regard it as a relatively low risk. There is no doubt, however, that diffuse fibrosing processes involving the lungs incur a much greater incidence of the subsequent development of a peripheral carcinoma. Thus, there is a much greater incidence of peripheral carcinoma of the lung in patients suffering from such conditions as asbestosis and idiopathic pulmonary fibrosis. Usually the tumour that arises is an adenocarcinoma, but occasionally squamous cell carcinomas or large cell anaplastic tumours may occur. Peripherally arising small cell carcinomas have been described but are exceptionally uncommon. Because peripheral adenocarcinomas are not related to smoking cigarettes, they used to be relatively more common in women. Now, however, with more women smoking this difference in pattern has largely been lost.

Large Cell Anaplastic Carcinoma

This is not a specific entity and represents a group of primary lung carcinomas that cannot be classified into the groups outlined above (Plate 4.1d). Most large cell

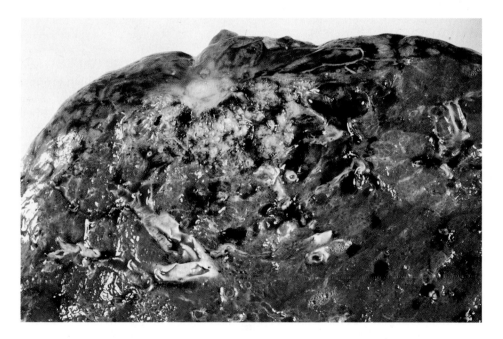

Plate 4.2   Scar carcinoma. The visceral pleura is seen at the top and is puckered into a central scar. Beneath the scar and radiating out into the subjacent lung tissue is whitish tumour tissue. Peripherally-arising scar cancers are usually adenocarcinomas, but other varieties may occur.

anaplastic carcinomas, therefore, represent tumours arising from the bronchial epithelium which have not differentiated sufficiently to allow them to be placed in either the squamous cell carcinoma or adenocarcinoma groups. The clinical behaviour of this group of tumours is similar to centrally arising adenocarcinomas and not
as good as well differentiated squamous cell carcinomas. They do not, however, behave nearly so aggressively as small cell carcinomas.

Metastatic Carcinoma

One problem that frequently confronts the pathologist, particularly with resection
specimens, is to establish whether a carcinoma is primary or secondary in type.
Although metastatic squamous carcinoma may occasionally mimic a bronchial
primary (e.g. metastatic from the uterine cervix), it is usually with adenocarcinoma
that this problem is encountered. Metastatic adenocarcinomas from various sites in
the body may mimic primary lung adenocarcinomas, particularly those arising
peripherally. In practice, the presence of a single deposit, an associated scar, or
endobronchial or bronchiolar dysplasia may help to make the diagnosis of a primary
neoplasm. However, even the lepidic pattern of spread of broncho-alveolar carcinoma
may be mimicked by metastatic tumours from the biliary tract and pancreas, and the
sometimes multicentric nature of this neoplasm compounds the problem.

HISTOLOGICAL DIAGNOSIS

The WHO2 classification is a practical one, relying on only a haematoxylin and eosin
(H/E) stained section and the skill of the observer to determine to which group a
lung carcinoma should be allocated. In the case of large cell tumours a mucin stain
is used in order to decide whether the tumour should be allocated to the large cell
anaplastic group (mucin negative) or to the adenocarcinoma group (solid carcinoma
with mucus formation: category 3d). If additional specialized techniques are used,
however the situation becomes much more complicated. The small cell group of
tumours are categorized ultrastructurally by the presence of numerous dense core
granules, but smaller numbers of these structures may also be seen in a fair proportion
of tumours classed by H/E staining as large cell anaplastic carcinomas. Even using
the straightforward WHO2 classification, a large proportion of lung cancers that
have been extensively sampled histologically will show more than one pattern of
differentiation and it is now accepted that with centrally arising lung cancers, some
degree of heterogeneity of differentiation is the norm rather than the exception.
This fact is acknowledged to some extent in the WHO2 classification with the provision
of a mixed group in the small cell carcinoma category (2c) — combined oat cell
carcinoma. Category 5 in the WHO2 classification is adenosquamous carcinoma and
this represents a tumour showing both squamous and adenocarcinomatous
differentiation.

   From a very basic, but practical, point of view, the histopathologist should be able
to tell his clinical colleagues whether or not the lung cancer that he has diagnosed is

of the small cell type or not. Thus from the point of view of clinical staging and management, a very simplified classification of primary lung cancer is into 'small cell carcinoma' and 'non-small cell carcinoma'. Even on very small amounts of often very traumatized material, the histopathologist is very good at making this distinction.

MACROSCOPIC APPEARANCES

The ability of lung cancer to arise both centrally from main or segmental bronchi and peripherally from bronchioles and alveoli, means that it is capable of giving rise to a wide variety of appearances (Plate 4.3).

The central or hilar types of tumour tend to invade the bronchial wall causing ulceration and narrowing of the lumen. This may result in haemoptysis or in bronchial obstruction. The tumour infiltrates along the bronchial walls, often in lymphatic vessels. Bronchial obstruction may result in lung collapse with or without retention ('lipid') pneumonia, secondary bronchopneumonia or lung abscess formation. A clinical presentation of 'unresolved' pneumonia or recurrent pneumonia is suggestive of an underlying neoplasm. The tumour may spread out from the bronchus into the adjacent lung parenchyma and lymphatic spread results in enlargement of the hilar lymph nodes. 'Lymphangitis carcinomatosa' is the term given to a lung cancer (or sometimes metastatic carcinoma — particularly from breast) which spreads extensively throughout the lung parenchyma via the perivascular and peribronchial lymphatic channels. Ultimately, widespread dissemination in this way results in an interstitial pattern of lung disease with reduced diffusion capacity and reduced lung compliance.

Involvement of the pleura by lung carcinoma may lead to a pleural effusion or pleurisy. The pericardium may be involved and lung cancer is the commonest tumour to metastasize to the heart. Extension of the tumour into the mediastinum may cause compression of the great vessels such as the superior vena cava or other structures such as the trachea. Involvement of the recurrent laryngeal nerve causes hoarseness.

Pancoast tumour is a primary lung carcinoma, usually of squamous type, which arises in the apex of the lung and spreads to the brachial plexus and the cervical sympathetic chain; the involvement of the latter results in the development of Horner's syndrome. It should be noted, however, that any infiltrative mass lesion occurring in the apices of the lung will give rise to similar results (Pancoast's syndrome) and need not necessarily be neoplastic.

The peripheral types of lung tumours often spread extensively throughout the lung tissue producing pneumonic like consolidation. The tumours then spread to the hilum and adjacent lymph nodes.

METASTATIC SPREAD

Although disseminated spread of lung cancer is seen most commonly with the small cell types, virtually all varieties may spread widely and the pattern of lymphatic and blood spread is identical for all the histological types. Thus, all may metastasize to

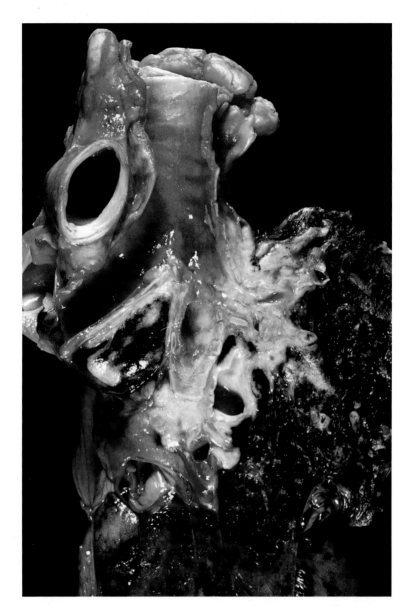

Plate 4.3 Centrally-arising lung cancer. This is carcinoma of the right lung seen from the posterior aspect. The right main stem bronchus and its branches are thickened and occluded by carcinoma. The heavily anthracotic lung is collapsed. The carina is widened and a mass of anthracotic and tumour-replaced lymph nodes are present in the tracheal bifurcation. The tumour has extended out into the mediastinum, and surrounds the aortic arch seen in cross section above the left main bronchus. The carcinoma was of large cell anaplastic type.

the peribronchial, paratracheal and mediastinal lymph nodes with later further extension to the lower cervical, upper abdominal and para-aortic lymph nodes.

Lung cancer characteristically spreads by the blood to the skeleton, the liver, the brain, the skin and the adrenal glands. It is the common metastatic tumour to involve the adrenal glands, and, at post mortem examination, metastatic spread to the adrenals is found in over 25% of cases. In the United Kingdom lung cancer is now the commonest cause of bilateral adrenal destruction (replacing tuberculosis) resulting in Addison's disease.

In cases of disseminated tumour, the distribution of lung cancer at autopsy is often highly characteristic, particularly if there is adrenal involvement, and may point to the presence of an undiagnosed primary lung cancer. This is particularly important with small cell tumours where the primary tumour may be extremely small. Small cell carcinoma may also occasionally present with obstructive jaundice due to massive enlargement of upper abdominal and peripancreatic lymph nodes. The primary carcinoma may remain undisclosed, and a diagnosis of primary pancreatic carcinoma may be made erroneously.

Lung cancer is one of the few malignant neoplasms which commonly spreads metastatically to the kidney and spleen. Apart from metastatic prostatic carcinoma, lung carcinoma (particularly the small cell type) is the commonest tumour to metastasize to the testis.

LESS COMMON TUMOURS

Carcinoid Tumour (see Chapter 13)

This is the most common benign tumour of the lung, accounting for about 1% to 2% of lung tumours. It characteristically occurs in an earlier age group and the tumour usually presents as a centrally arising polypoid mass occluding a bronchus (Plates 4.4a and 4.4b). Carcinoid tumours are benign neuroendocrine tumours, essentially the benign counterpart of the small cell carcinoma. Histologically, they resemble carcinoid tumours elsewhere in the body (Plate 4.5), and surgical resection is usually curative. Occasionally these tumours may be multicentric and they may also occasionally metastasise to local lymph nodes. Very rarely, distant metastases from these tumours, particularly to the liver, may result in the carcinoid syndrome or, very rarely, in Cushing's syndrome.

The above description relates to the usual or so-called 'classical' carcinoid tumour. Less commonly tumours may arise in the lung which resemble classical carcinoids in their histological appearance but which consist of larger, often spindle cells, with much more mitotic activity. These tumours, however, show the same ultrastructural features as carcinoid tumours and are termed 'atypical carcinoid tumours'. It is most important that the atypical carcinoid tumour is distinguished from the large cell anaplastic group and particularly from the intermediate cell type of small cell carcinoma. Atypical carcinoids may be regarded as a 'half-way house' between the

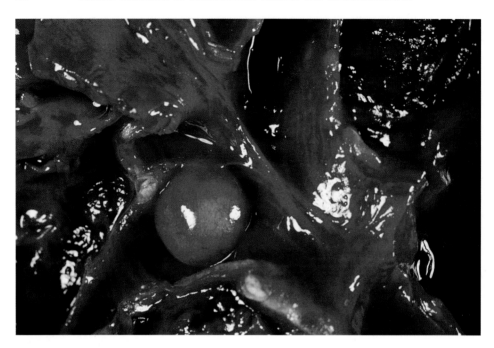

Plate 4.4a   Carcinoid tumour. A lobectomy specimen showing a polypoid tumour in a main bronchus. Note the smooth surface indicating that the bronchial epithelium is intact and the tumour is submucosal.

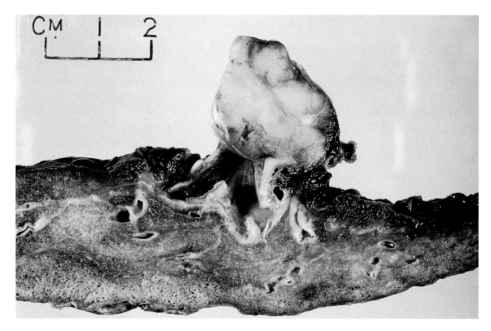

Plate 4.4b   Carcinoid tumour. The same specimen as Plate 4.4a, now fixed and bisected. The tumour nodule is seen occluding the bronchus, the lobe is collapsed and the air passages contain purulent mucus.

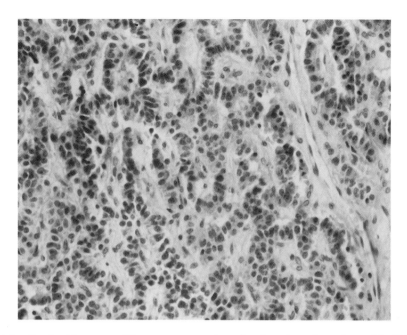

Plate 4.5 Carcinoid tumour. The tumour consists of trabeculae of regular epithelial cells. There are no mitotic figures. The appearances are identical to those of carcinoid tumours elsewhere in the body.

relatively benign carcinoid tumour of classical type and small cell carcinoma. The prognosis is not as good as the former, but very much better than the latter.

Bronchial Gland Tumours

These are all rare; they arise from the bronchial glands and show differentiation patterns similar to those seen in salivary gland tumours. The common patterns are adenoid cystic carcinoma and mucoepidermoid carcinoma. Bronchial gland tumours show very variable rates of growth and some are relatively benign (the so-called 'bronchial adenoma' group) but at the other end of the spectrum a behaviour pattern similar to that of centrally arising adenocarcinoma is not unusual.

Hamartoma

Hamartomas of the lung are not uncommon. They tend to arise peripherally and are seen as 'coin' lesions on chest X-rays. They consist of masses of bronchial epithelium and hyaline cartilage together with other mesenchymal elements. Their main importance is in the differential diagnosis of coin lesions of the lung, but pulmonary hamartomas may grow in adult life and may behave more aggressively than their name might suggest.

Carcinosarcoma

These tumours arise infrequently in the lung. They consist of a mixture of epithelial and mesenchymal elements and usually present as polypoid endobronchial growths; they spread quickly and have usually metastasized by the time of diagnosis. Very rarely in children and young adults, a type of carcinosarcoma may arise which contains embryonal elements. These tumours are called pulmonary blastomas and carry a poor prognosis.

Mesenchymal tumours

Rarely, benign and malignant mesenchymal tumours may arise in the lung. Thus, simple tumours such as lipomas may present 'mass lesion' effects. Simple leiomyomas of the lung do occur, but this diagnosis should be treated with suspicion particularly in females where metastatic smooth muscle tumours from the corpus uteri should be considered. Sarcomas are very uncommon.

Lymphoma

Primary non-Hodgkin's lymphoma may arise in the lung but is uncommon. It may be very indolent; some examples were previously known as pseudolymphomas and were confused with lymphocytic interstitial pneumonitis (LIP). Some of these tumours may arise from mucosa-associated lymphoid tissue (MALT) and reflect the behaviour of MALT lymphomas in other parts of the body. Many authorities would argue that pseudolymphoma, as an entity, does not exist and that all these tumours are examples of low-grade MALT lymphomas. High-grade non-Hodgkin's lymphomas and, less commonly, Hodgkin's disease may also spread metastatically to involve the lung.

PLEURAL TUMOURS

Pleural Fibroma

This uncommon tumour is thought to arise from sub-serosal multipotential mesothelial cells. It usually arises from the parietal pleura and may be very large. Fibromas form a polypoid mass within the thoracic cavity and may cause pressure effects on the lungs or heart. Although usually benign, some of these tumours (about 25%) may grow fairly rapidly and may even metastasize. Some may be associated with rheumatoid-like arthropathy, which resolves once the tumour has been resected, and others with fever or isolated hypoglycaemia. This tumour is sometimes known as 'benign mesothelioma' or 'local mesothelioma'.

Pleural Plaques

White fibrous pleural plaques which are composed of hyalinized and relatively acellular collagen may be found on the parietal pleura and over the parietal pericardium and diaphragm in patients who have been exposed to asbestos. The presence of pleural plaques which, because of secondary dystrophic calcification, may be seen on chest X-ray or CAT scanning, is good evidence of exposure to asbestos, but they do not in themselves indicate asbestos-related disease such as diffuse pleural fibrosis, asbestosis or asbestos-related tumour.

Malignant Mesothelioma (see Chapter 14)

The incidence of this tumour in any community is directly proportional to asbestos exposure, particularly exposure to the amphibole or straight fibre varieties (blue asbestos, crocidolite, and brown asbestos, amosite). Chrysotile, the only common form of serpentine asbestos, although implicated in the pathogenesis of asbestosis, is not regarded as being a significant cause of mesothelioma because the curly fibres do not reach the periphery of the lung nor therefore the pleura. In the United Kingdom some 90% of malignant mesotheliomas are clearly associated with asbestos exposure. Although at one time it was considered to be a rare tumour, the long latent period of between 20 and 40 years has meant that increasing numbers of cases are being diagnosed. In the United Kingdom the number of patients presenting with this tumour may continue to increase well into the next century.

Malignant mesothelioma may exist in either an epithelial form which resembles adenocarcinoma or a mesenchymal form, the appearance of which is that of a spindle-celled sarcoma. These forms may exist separately or in combination (mixed tumours). Mesotheliomas do not tend to invade the lung parenchyma but grow round the pleural space and into the chest wall (Plate 4.6). The tumour encases the lung, compressing it and causing atelectasis. Because of its propensity for chest-wall invasion, this neoplasm may seed out through biopsy or surgical incisions or even needle biopsy tracts. Although mesothelioma usually kills by local growth and complications, it does metastasize, having the same pattern of metastatic spread as bronchial carcinoma. Metastatic spread is present in over 50% of cases of mesothelioma at post mortem.

Desmoplastic mesothelioma is a variant that produces large amounts of fibrous tissue, the malignant cells themselves being difficult to identify in a mass of collagen. This type of tumour is very difficult to diagnose even by open biopsy and occasionally even post mortem examination may fail to completely distinguish this tumour from a reactive fibrous pleurisy.

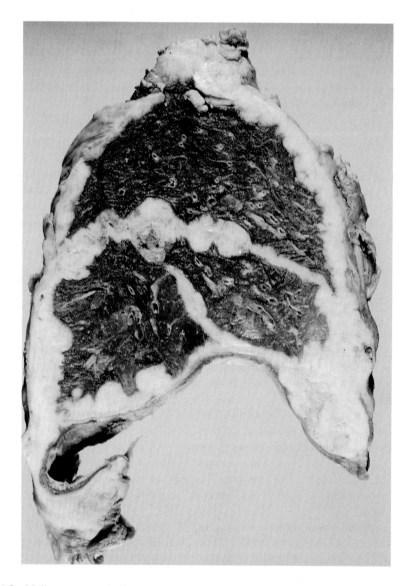

Plate 4.6   Malignant mesothelioma. The tumour has grown round the pleural space and into the interlobar fissures. The diaphragm is seen attached at the bottom and the tumour is invading the chest wall. The lung is collapsed.

KEY POINTS

- There are four main types of bronchial carcinoma: squamous cell, adenocarcinoma, large cell anaplastic and small cell anaplastic.
- The most important distinction that the pathologist must make for the clinician is between small cell carcinoma and the others.
- Most carcinomas arise "centrally" from main and segmental bronchi and only 20% arise "peripherally" from the lung parenchyma.
- Less common lung tumours include carcinoid and brochial gland tumours, hamartomas, carcinosarcomas, mesenchymal tumours and lymphomas.
- The most important pleural tumour is malignant mesothelioma, which is associated with asbestos exposure.

REFERENCES

1. World Health Organization. (1967) Histological typing of lung tumours. *International histological classification of tumours. No. 1.* 1st edn. Geneva: WHO.
2. World Health Organisation. (1981) Histological typing of lung tumours. *International histological classification of tumours. No. 1.* 2nd edn. Geneva: WHO.
3. Burnett R.A., Beck J.S., Howatson S.R., Lee F.D., Lessells A.M., McLaren K.M., Ogston S., Robertson A.J., Simpson J.G., Smith G.D., Tavadia H.B., Walker F. (1994) Observer variability in histopathological reporting of malignant bronchial biopsy specimens. *J. Clin. Pathol.* **47**, 711–713.

FURTHER READING

Lamb D. (1987) *Lung Cancer and its Classification.* In *Recent Advances in Histopathology* **13**, edited by Anthony P.P., MacSween R.N.M. pp. 45–59. Edinburgh: Churchill Livingstone.
Santona M.J. (Ed) (1994) Pathology of Pulmonary Disease Chapters 46–61. Philadelphia: J.B. Lippiniott Company.
Jones J.S.P. (Ed) (1987) *Pathology of the Mesothelium.* London: Springer-Verlag.

5 NON-SMALL CELL LUNG CANCER: NON-SURGICAL MANAGEMENT

For clinical purposes, patients with lung cancer who have tumours with squamous cell, adenocarcinoma, or large cell anaplastic histology are usually considered together using the rather cumbersome term non-small cell lung cancer (NSCLC). This is because for practical purposes they are managed in the same way. There may be slight differences in the prognosis or the pattern of metastasis (brain metastases seem to be more frequent in patients with adenocarcinoma) but at the moment these are not enough to change the general principles of management.

The most important point is that the treatment of choice for these patients is primary surgery. Although only a minority (perhaps 25%) will have resectable disease, every effort should be made as soon as possible to establish whether or not they are operable. The surgical management is described fully in Chapter 6, and in this chapter we will concentrate on the non-surgical treatment options.

PROGNOSTIC FACTORS

It is important to try to make some assessment of the patient's likely prognosis when they are first seen and decisions about treatment have to be made. This assessment will obviously never be a precise indicator of the eventual course of the disease but will give some general guidelines.

There have been attempts to combine important prognostic factors, variously weighted for their importance, to produce prognostic indices. Although these are interesting research tools, it is not clear whether they offer advantage over assessment by an experienced clinician. The factors discussed below seem to be the most significant.

Stage

The stage of disease at presentation is the most important prognostic factor. The most widely used staging system is the New International System (Mountain, 1986), which is summarized in Table 5.1.

One difficulty with the use of this staging system is that it is very dependent on accurate determination of whether or not intrathoracic lymph nodes are involved by tumour. This is sometimes obvious on plain X-ray or CT scan when there is gross enlargement of nodes, but the detection of microscopic involvement requires invasive surgical investigation. This is discussed further in Chapter 6, as is the value of screening investigations for metastatic disease.

For many patients, however, surgery is not an option and accurate surgical staging is not appropriate and so it is only possible to guess whether the disease is Stage IIIA or IIIB. This may not be important in most instances, but is of great relevance in

Table 5.1   TNM STAGING OF LUNG CANCER (New International Staging System).

T1	Tumour 3 cm or less in greatest dimension, but not in main bronchus.
T2	Tumour more than 3 cm in greatest dimension, **or** involving main bronchus, 2 cm or more distal to carina, **or** invading visceral pleura, **or** associated with atelectasis or obstructive pneumonitis, not involving the whole lung.
T3	Tumour of any size, directly invading chest wall, diaphragm, mediastinal pleura or parietal pericardium; **or** in a main bronchus, less than 2 cm from, but not involving, the carina; **or** associated with atelectasis or obstructive pneumonitis of the whole lung.
T4	Tumour of any size invading mediastinum, heart, great vessels, trachea, oesophagus, vertebral body or carina; **or** associated with malignant pleural effusion.
NX	Regional lymph nodes cannot be assessed.
N0	No regional lymph nodes metastasis.
N1	Metastasis to ipsilateral peribronchial and/or hilar lymph nodes.
N2	Metastasis to ipsilateral mediastinal and/or subcarinal lymph nodes.
N3	Metastasis to contralateral mediastinal or hilar lymph nodes, or scalene or supraclavicular lymph nodes.
M0	No distant metastasis.
M1	Distant metastasis.

Stage Grouping

Stage I	T1 or T2 N0 M0
Stage II	T1 or T2 N1 M0
Stage IIIA	T3 or N2 M0
Stage IIIB	T4 or N3 M0
Stage IV	M1

trials of radical radiotherapy alone or in combination with chemotherapy. For patients receiving palliative radiotherapy, the only relevant staging is an assessment of whether they have 'limited' disease, confined to one hemithorax, or 'extensive' disease with metastases beyond the chest (see below).

Performance Status

Performance status (PS) is a 'crude' general assessment of the patient's general fitness. The most commonly used scale is the World Health Organization (WHO) PS scale shown in Table 5.2.

Despite being a very subjective, superficial assessment, PS is a remarkably good predictor of outcome and, in most multivariate analyses of survival, emerges as a strong prognostic factor. As well as being an important tool in all clinical trials it is

Table 5.2   WHO Performance Status scale.

Score	Status
0	Normal activity without restriction
1	Strenuous activity restricted, can do light work
2	In bed for less than 50% of waking hours, can do light work
3	In bed for more than 50% of waking hours, limited self-care
4	Confined to bed or chair, no self-care, completely disabled

useful in the clinical management of patients. It is good practice to record PS when the patient is first seen, because it will sometimes influence important decisions about treatment and will give a fairly repeatable assessment of general fitness that can be monitored with time.

One slight problem with the use of the WHO PS scale in patients with NSCLC is the fact that the assessment is essentially one of functional capability. Many patients are limited partly by their respiratory function, particularly if they have underlying chronic lung disease, and this may reduce their PS to a level that is not entirely consistent with their actual tumour burden. It is therefore also worth recording their respiratory status (RS), even if formal pulmonary function tests are not done. A useful scale is the Medical Research Council RS scale (Table 5.3).

Weight Loss

Weight loss is another important prognostic factor. Lung cancer of all types is particularly associated with anorexia and cachexia. It is not necessarily a sign of metastatic disease, and some patients with truly localized tumours can lose weight. It is therefore important to weigh patients at all their clinic visits and to make some assessment of the amount they have lost in the six months before first being seen.

The problem of anorexia and cachexia is discussed further in Chapter 10.

Table 5.3   MRC Respiratory Status scale.

Score	Status
0	Climbs hills or stairs without dyspnoea
1	Walks any distance on the flat without dyspnoea
2	Walks over 100 m without dyspnoea
3	Dyspnoea on walking 100 m or less
4	Dyspnoea at rest

Metastases

Although deciding whether metastases are present or not is part of the staging process, it is worth emphasizing the important prognostic significance of obvious metastatic disease at presentation. From 70% to 80% of patients with metastases will die within six months and almost all within a year. Even the presence of an elevated alkaline phosphatase result on routine biochemical screening conveys a worse prognosis in the absence of overt liver or bone metastases.

Histology

In some surgical series, the precise histology does seem to have prognostic significance, patients with adenocarcinoma appearing to do worse than those with other types of NSCLC. In particular there seems to be higher incidence of relapse with brain metastases. For patients with more advanced disease, however, precise histology does not seem to be a major prognostic factor.

MANAGEMENT POLICIES

Surgery is the treatment of choice for patients with NSCLC and the only treatment that is associated with a significant chance of long-term survival (see Chapter 6). Although every effort should be made to ensure that potential patients are operated on, it is wrong to let emotion cloud judgement about younger patients and refer them for surgery when there is good evidence that they are inoperable. An unnecessary thoracotomy is a failure of management and may leave a patient not only with the problems of post-operative chest-wall pain, but also the psychological problems of disappointment at losing a chance of cure.

Radiotherapy is the next best option for treatment. There is a group of patients who are likely to benefit from high-dose, radical radiotherapy, and a small proportion may be long-term survivors. As is discussed below, attitudes to radical radiotherapy vary considerably from centre to centre, which can be confusing for the non-specialist and lead to patients who potentially might benefit not being referred. Any patient who is reasonably fit but inoperable for medical reasons (e.g. moderately poor lung function or heart disease) should at least be considered for radical radiotherapy, as should any patient without metastatic disease and a Pancoast tumour or small volume disease involving trachea, proximal main-stem bronchi or chest wall.

Palliative radiotherapy is certainly effective in controlling the symptoms of lung cancer and need not be associated with great morbidity. All symptomatic patients should be considered for treatment.

In the United Kingdom chemotherapy is not considered to be a routine treatment for most patients with NSCLC, though its place is being reassessed. With a few exceptions, its use should at the moment be restricted to the context of clinical trials.

There are a number of clinical problems associated with advanced lung cancer and metastatic disease, which all need skilled and appropriate management. These are discussed in Chapters 8, 9 and 10.

RADICAL RADIOTHERAPY: WHAT IS IT?

The role of radical radiotherapy in the management of NSCLC is a subject that is rather confusing to the non-specialist. There seem to be widely held contradictory views about its appropriateness and, until recently, few good research studies to help an objective appraisal.

To a radiation oncologist 'radical' treatment means treatment to a dose that has a reasonable chance of producing local control of the tumour, and may be associated with a finite, though not excessive, risk of short- and long-term morbidity. A problem is that, in the case of lung cancer, different radiation oncologists may have very different ideas of what constitutes an appropriate radical treatment.

The differences hinge on three important variables: dose, duration of treatment, and volume treated. It is a fundamental principle of radiobiology that the dose needed to control a particular tumour increases the longer the time over which the treatment is given, and so a dose of 60 Gray (Gy) given over six weeks is probably equivalent to 55 Gy in four weeks or 50 Gy in three weeks. But the risk of late tissue damage from radiotherapy (e.g. lung fibrosis, oesophageal stenosis, spinal cord damage) increases the larger the individual fractions of treatment are. This means that the shorter treatments can only be given to small volumes of the patient, whereas the more prolonged treatments can safely be given to larger volumes.

The different philosophies of treatment fall into three groups which are discussed below.

Small Volume/Short Time

A typical treatment of this type would be a dose of 50 Gy (minimum tumour dose) given in 15 fractions over three weeks to a volume that does not exceed $8 \times 8 \times 8$ cm. This means that only relatively small primary tumours can be treated and inherent in this philosophy is the belief that patients with larger tumours or mediastinal node involvement are incurable. The only patients treated are those with T1N0 or T2N0 tumours who are medically unfit for surgery, or those with small T3N0 tumours, inoperable because of direct mediastinal or possibly chest wall involvement.

Intermediate Volume/Intermediate Time

A typical treatment of this type would be a dose of 50–55 Gy (minimum tumour dose) given in 20 fractions over 4 weeks to a volume up to $10 \times 12 \times 10$ cm. This volume would include larger tumours and also, if the primary was proximal, involved mediastinal nodes. It would not include the whole mediastinum. A variant of this is a 'split course' treatment in which the patient is given 30 Gy in two weeks, reviewed a month later and, if still well with evidence of response and no metastatic disease, gets a further 20 Gy in 10 fractions.

Shrinking Volume/Long Time

This policy involves treating the patient with so called 'conventional' fractions of 2 Gy daily, giving a total dose of 60–70 Gy (minimum tumour dose) over six or seven weeks. A wide area covering mediastinal and even supraclavicular fossa lymph nodes is treated to start with, on the assumption that there may be micrometastatic disease. After 40–45 Gy the treatment is replanned to cover only the area of macroscopic disease.

These policies of treatment are clearly quite different in their complexity, use of resources and above all in the kind of patients who are suitable. The first policy is the most selective and only patients with a small volume of disease and minimal mediastinal involvement will be selected, whereas patients with quite bulky tumours and extensive mediastinal spread (N2 disease) may be treated with the third policy. This in turn may well affect the possible outcome in terms of disease control.

There is a quite widely held view in the United Kingdom that radical radiotherapy is of no benefit and that inoperable patients should either get palliative radiotherapy or no treatment if asymptomatic. So, what is the evidence to support the use of radical radiotherapy? It has to be said that it is not strong and is entirely circumstantial.

The only randomized study to compare 'radical' with palliative radiotherapy was carried out by the Veterans Administration in the USA in the 1960s.[1] It showed only a modest benefit, but the doses and techniques of radiotherapy were not comparable to modern radical radiotherapy and patients with SCLC were included. There has been no randomized study in the modern era to investigate this question.

The circumstantial evidence, from studies comparing different dose schedules, is that there is a correlation between increasing dose and better survival. Also most studies of radical radiotherapy give broadly similar survival figures with a small but consistent number of long-term (five-year) survivors.

RADICAL RADIOTHERAPY: HOW TO DO IT

We believe that radical radiotherapy does have a place in the management of selected patients with NSCLC, and will briefly describe our selection policy, planning and treatment techniques, the technical problems and possible morbidity.

Patient Selection

The patients should be fit (PS 0, 1 or 2) with minimal (<5%) weight loss and no evidence of metastatic disease on clinical examination, biochemical screening and liver ultrasound (or CT scan). The primary tumour and any detectable mediastinal spread should be encompassable in a volume no greater than $10 \times 12 \times 10$ cm. They need to have adequate respiratory reserve to cope with the loss of 25–30% of the lung function. An FEV1 of less than 50% of predicted is a usual cut-off but some patients with a lower figure may cope with a small volume treatment of a peripheral tumour. Severe ischaemic heart disease is not a contraindication.

It is a counsel of perfection to have a histological diagnosis before embarking on radical radiotherapy, but certainly it is essential for all clinical trials. There are quite a number of patients with small peripheral tumours and no histology obtained at bronchoscopy who are inoperable for medical reasons (poor lung function, ischaemic heart disease etc.) but who might be suitable for radical radiotherapy. It may be possible to obtain cytology by needle biopsy but this can be traumatic and there is the risk of pneumothorax. It may then be necessary to treat them on the basis of clinical likelihood, and any patient with significant risk factors and a typical enlarging mass on chest X-ray should be considered.

Planning Technique

Whenever possible the treatment should be planned using a CT system, as the information from plain X-ray pictures is not adequate in most cases. The patients should be supine with their arms above their head and it may be helpful to use a simple immobilization device to maintain the position accurately.

The target volume should be defined leaving a margin of 2 cm around the macroscopic tumour to allow for microscopic spread, inaccuracies in positioning and respiratory movement. There is often a real problem in identifying the margins of tumour on CT scans accurately, especially when there is adjacent collapse and consolidation of the lung or mediastinal invasion, and arbitrary decisions may have to be made. If available, information from bronchoscopy, mediastinoscopy or thoracotomy can be helpful.

Once the beam arrangements have been planned, they need to be checked on the simulator and, ideally with "port" films at the first treatment.

Treatment Technique and Dose

The usual technique for treatment of central tumours is a three-field arrangement of beams as shown in Figure 5.1. This allows for a good dose distribution over the target volume but avoids the spinal cord. The ipsilateral lung obviously gets quite a high-dose and parts of the contralateral lung may get 40–50% doses. If there is a significant risk of lung damage it should be possible to start the treatment with opposed fields (Figure 5.2) and then go on to a three-field arrangement for the second half of the course. Although this will reduce the amount of lung irradiated, care is needed with the spinal cord which will receive the full tumour dose during the first phase of treatment.

Care is also needed with the spinal cord dose at the upper end of the treatment volume. The upper part of the thoracic cord tends to come anteriorly and may come close to or into the high-dose volume. It should be possible to shield the upper part

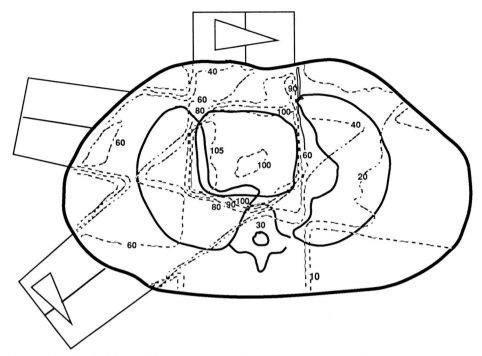

Figure 5.1   Typical three-field radiotherapy plan for treating a central tumour.

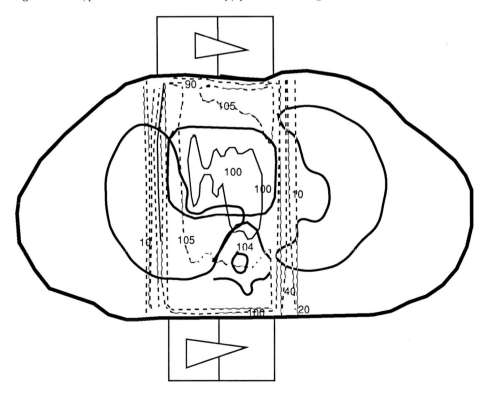

Figure 5.2   Typical opposed-field radiotherapy plan for treating a central tumour.

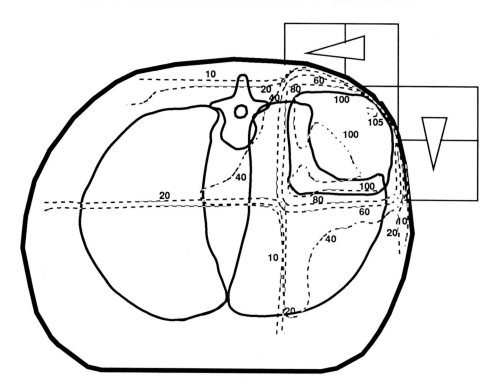

Figure 5.3   Typical two field ('wedge-pair') radiotherapy plan for treating a small peripheral tumour.

of the cord from the postero-lateral field and so reduce the dose to acceptable levels (i.e. below 44 to 46 Gy).

One can sometimes reduce the amount of normal lung irradiated by shielding areas (especially on the anterior field) that come into the high-dose volume but that do not need to be treated.

Small peripheral tumours, especially those abutting or invading the chest wall, may be best treated with a pair of wedged fields (Figure 5.3) and it may be possible to plan such treatments using orthogonal X-rays rather than a CT scan.

The dose we use is 52 to 55 Gy in 20 fractions over four weeks. This is a compromise between the more prolonged 6 week treatment, that is universal in the United States and most of Europe, and the short 15-fraction regimen. Provided the spinal cord dose is safe and the volume of normal lung treated is kept to a minimum, there are no critical structures in the volume that dictate the use of 2 Gy fractions. The use of the 15-fraction regimen requires more rigorous patient selection and care in keeping the volume small.

'Split course' regimens, though attractive from a practical point of view, have been shown in other sites to be less effective than continuous treatment, probably because tumour repopulation can occur during the break from treatment.

RADICAL RADIOTHERAPY: SIDE EFFECTS

Systemic

Radical radiotherapy to the chest is usually well tolerated. General tiredness is frequent but nausea and vomiting unusual.

Oesophagitis

When the oesophagus is in the high-dose volume, as it almost always is when central tumours are treated, the patient will develop radiation oesophagitis in about the third week. This is due to acute radiation damage to the epithelium causing denudation of the epithelial surface and an inflammatory mucositis. It can usually be managed with topical analgesics (e.g. Mucaine) and a semi-solid diet and it is very unusual for it to be severe enough for patients to be admitted for nasogastric feeding. Because it is due to radiation damage it does not respond to antacids or other conventional measures for oesophagitis, though it is made worse by acid reflux and, in patients with known reflux oesophagitis, conventional treatment should be continued.

Radiation oesophagitis usually settles spontaneously two or three weeks after radiotherapy finishes. Occasionally it can be persistent and, if so, other problems such as acid reflux or oesophageal thrush should be considered.

Very rarely, patients may get oesophageal stenosis as a late effect of radiation some years after radiotherapy. This is unusual and can usually be treated adequately by regular bouginage.

Radiation Pneumonitis

Radiation pneumonitis occurs whenever parts of the lung receive doses above 20 Gy and is probably due to radiation damage to the Type II pneumocytes in the alveoli. X-ray changes are universal, but the clinical syndrome only occurs in a minority of patients, perhaps 10 or 20%.

The classic symptoms are of a dry, unproductive cough, increasing dyspnoea and slight wheeze coming on six to eight weeks after radiotherapy. The chest X-ray shows an area of diffuse nodular shadowing within the area of lung that received the high-dose. This period of 'acute pneumonitis' lasts for three to four weeks and then resolves. It is usual to give corticosteroids (e.g. prednisolone 30 mg daily) to symptomatic patients but it is not clear whether or not this actually influences the course of the condition.

After six to nine months pulmonary fibrosis will eventually occur in the high-dose area as a permanent change. How disabling this will be for the patient will depend on their respiratory reserve before treatment and the care with which the treatment was initially planned.

Radiation Myelitis

Provided that attention is paid to the dose to the spinal cord throughout its length and it does not exceed 46 Gy in 2 Gy fractions, radiation myelitis should not be a problem. If a patient does subsequently develop symptoms and signs of spinal cord damage, investigation for other causes should be carried out before attributing it to the radiotherapy.

RADICAL RADIOTHERAPY: RESULTS

What results can one expect from putting patients through a course of radical radiotherapy? This depends first of all on the patients selected for treatment. A number of series of patients with T1N0 and T2N0 tumours treated with radical radiotherapy rather than surgery (because of intercurrent medical problems, age or refusal) have been described. The two-year survival for these patients is around 50% and the five-year survival 20 to 30%. This of course does not compare well with surgical series which report five-year survival figures of 50 to 60% for patients at a similar stage, but it must be remembered that the patients getting radiotherapy have a higher risk of intercurrent death and may have been turned down for surgery because of their other medical problems.

The results of radical radiotherapy for patients with more advanced local disease are less good. Most published series report a median survival of around 10 months, a two-year survival of 15 to 20% and a five-year survival of about 5% (Figure 5.4).

RADICAL RADIOTHERAPY: THE FUTURE

The results of radical radiotherapy for small tumours are good enough to justify its continued use for this selected group of patients. The results for patients with more bulky disease are clearly disappointing and call its routine use into question, particularly when everyone has anecdotal experience of patients surviving for five years after palliative radiotherapy, and some series of patients with good performance status treated with palliative radiotherapy have been reported with two-year survival figures that are not much less than those quoted above. There is therefore a place for a randomized trial comparing radical with palliative radiotherapy in patients with locally advanced tumours but it seems unlikely that this trial will ever take place. Instead new ideas are being tested.

There are two problems in treating locally advanced NSCLC. First there is the problem of local control and it is clear that the kind of doses that are currently used for radical radiotherapy do not produce local control in more than 30 to 40% of patients with bulky disease. Increasing the dose probably increases morbidity, without an increase in overall survival.

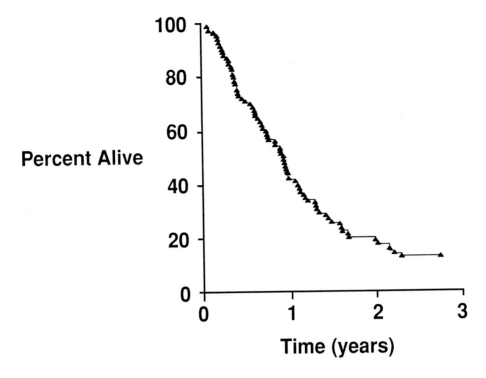

Figure 5.4   Actuarial survival of 95 patients with NSCLC treated with radical radiotherapy in Glasgow.

Three strategies are now being used to improve local control: combining chemotherapy with radiotherapy (see below), giving hyperfractionated (two or three times a day) radiotherapy and 'conformal' radiotherapy. There are theoretical reasons why hyperfractionation may improve local control and some promising initial results have been published. A major randomized study is underway in the United Kingdom at the moment to test its efficacy and until it is complete, hyperfractionation can only be regarded as experimental. New and sophisticated planning, and radiotherapy treatment systems are allowing the target volume to be shaped in three dimensions to fit more accurately to the tumour. With this 'conformal' radiotherapy it is theoretically possible to reduce the volume of normal tissue treated and therefore to increase the tumour dose without an increase in morbidity. Once again the value of this approach, which is expensive and time consuming, has not been established.

The second major problem is that of metastatic disease. Most patients will develop metastatic disease eventually whether or not their local disease is controlled. Again, the only chance of preventing this is by a combination of treatment with chemotherapy and radiotherapy (see below).

POST-OPERATIVE RADIOTHERAPY

There are two situations when radical radiotherapy might be considered after tumour resection. The first is when the margins of excision are not clear and microscopic tumour is found extending to the resection margin, or the surgeon is aware that macroscopic disease has been left behind. This is most likely to occur when tumours extend to and infiltrate the pleura and chest wall. In this situation it is probably worthwhile giving radical radiotherapy to a localized volume covering the area at risk. It is very helpful if the surgeon has left metal clips marking the areas of doubt.

The second situation is when, at surgery or histological examination, patients are found to have hilar or mediastinal lymph node involvement. There is evidence that post-operative radiotherapy increases local control in this situation, and one recent randomized trial has suggested that there may be a survival benefit for patients with N2 disease.[2]

PANCOAST TUMOURS

Patients with Pancoast or superior sulcus tumours constitute a separate group. The tumours arise in the lung apex, are usually squamous and tend to infiltrate locally into the brachial plexus, mediastinum and adjacent vertebral body and ribs before metastasizing.

Typically they are difficult to diagnose, and the patient may give a long history of increasing shoulder and arm pain before the diagnosis is established. By that time they often have signs of local extension, such as ipsilateral Horner's syndrome or neurological signs in the arm and hand, and there may be radiological evidence of rib destruction. Bronchoscopy is usually unhelpful and histological confirmation rarely obtained. It may be possible to get a needle biopsy but approaches to this area are difficult, and the diagnosis is not often in doubt.

The treatment of choice is probably a combination of surgery and radiotherapy, the most usual recommendation being pre-operative radiotherapy to a dose of 40 Gy, surgery and more radiotherapy to a total of 60 Gy. There is, however, no clear evidence from randomized controlled trials to show that this approach is better than radical radiotherapy alone.

Unfortunately, most patients are inoperable at the time of presentation because of the extent of local disease and they should be treated with radical radiotherapy unless there is evidence of metastatic disease or their general condition is too poor. Our technique is to use parallel opposed, wedged fields covering the obvious tumour, cervico-axillary canal and adjacent vertebral bodies up to spinal cord tolerance (34–37 Gy in 13 or 14 fractions) and then shrink the field in order to come off the spinal cord and give a total of 52–55 Gy (depending on tumour volume) in 20 fractions.

Most patients report an improvement in their pain but many do have persistent pain of neuropathic type even when the tumour is apparently controlled, and they may need other measures (see Chapter 10). The dose described above may be greater than tolerance for the nerve roots of the brachial plexus, and any long-term survivors do run the risk of radiation neuropathy. This risk is, however, worth taking in the interests of local disease control.

PALLIATIVE RADIOTHERAPY

Unfortunately, only a small proportion (5 to 10%) of inoperable patients with NSCLC will be suitable for radical radiotherapy. The remainder should be considered for palliative radiotherapy.

Indications

Any patient with symptoms directly attributable to their tumour should get palliative radiotherapy unless their general condition and prognosis is so poor that they are unlikely to survive more than a few days. In particular, those with haemoptysis, chest pain and cough are likely to benefit. Dyspnoea is a symptom that tends to respond less well, probably because many patients have underlying lung disease or because, if the dyspnoea is due to lung collapse and consolidation rather than just airway obstruction, the lung may not re-expand fully even if the tumour shrinks. Those with stridor and superior vena cava obstruction also need to be treated fairly urgently (see Chapter 10).

Techniques

The technique for palliative radiotherapy should be kept as simple as possible. Parallel opposed megavoltage fields are almost always used, with a volume that covers the obvious sites of disease that are causing symptoms. It is often helpful to have the bronchoscopy report as well as a chest X-ray when planning treatment, but it is generally better to be generous with the field sizes to cover possible areas of involvement. It is sometimes quite difficult to be sure of the tumour extent when there is major lung collapse and consolidation and often decisions about the margins have to be fairly arbitrary.

Until recently, the most usual doses for palliative radiotherapy were 30 Gy in 10 fractions or 20 Gy in 5 fractions. Two recent Medical Research Council (MRC) trials[3, 4] have shown that shorter schedules are just as effective and can reduce the number of visits for the patient. Based on the results of these trials we would now recommend that patients with poor performance status and obvious metastatic disease should be treated with a single fraction of 10 Gy, and fitter patients should get 17 Gy in two fractions a week apart with spinal cord shielding for the second fraction.

There has been a tendency to treat the fitter patients, particularly those with localized disease or pain from chest wall involvement with a slightly higher dose such as 36 Gy or 39 Gy in 12 or 13 fractions. This policy was recently tested in another MRC trial by comparison with giving 17 Gy in two fractions. Interestingly, the preliminary results of this study suggest that although the palliative benefits in terms of symptom control are similar, there appears to be a small, but significant, survival benefit from the higher dose treatment. Until the full results are available from longer follow-up, however, it is not possible to recommend this policy as a routine.

There is some debate as to whether patients who have inoperable NSCLC but are asymptomatic should be treated with palliative radiotherapy at the time of diagnosis or should only be treated if and when they become symptomatic. Certainly some patients die from either metastases or intercurrent disease before they become significantly symptomatic, but it is possible that early radiotherapy may delay the onset of local symptoms or possibly even (especially in the light of the preliminary results of the MRC study alluded to above) improve survival. This question is being tested in a current MRC trial and it is not possible to make any recommendations at the moment.

Side Effects

General

Tiredness and some general malaise are common side effects of palliative radiotherapy to the chest, but nausea and vomiting are uncommon. The large-fraction, shorter schedules are generally well tolerated by the patients and there seems to be no greater incidence of these side effects than with longer schedules.

Chest pain and rigors

Some patients (perhaps 20–30%) experience chest pain, sweats and rigors sometime during the first 24 hours after treatment, usually within two or three hours, after 8.5 Gy or 10 Gy treatments to the chest. These can occasionally be quite severe though usually lasting no more than 30 minutes, and it is perhaps worthwhile warning patients of these problems and reassuring them that they are not serious. The cause of these symptoms is unclear.

Oesophagitis

Radiation oesophagitis is dose-related and so should be less of a problem with palliative regimens than with radical radiotherapy. In fact the 10 Gy regimen seems to result in hardly any oesophagitis.

After 17 Gy in two fractions, symptoms develop 10 to 12 days after the first fraction and last about a week. They should be managed with topical analgesics such as Mucaine which should be given to patients to take away with them after the second fraction.

Radiation myelitis

One area for concern with the 17 Gy regimen has been that occasional patients seem to have developed paraplegia due to radiation myelitis at 9 to 12 months after treatment. The risk in patients who survive to 18 months may be as high as 5%, but the overall incidence seems to be low (less than 1%) because so few patients survive to the time of risk.

Our policy has been to shield the spinal cord from the posterior field only (1cm lead strip along the spine) for the second fraction, especially if the patient is relatively fit and might have a better prognosis. This does reduce the central dose in the midline from 17 Gy to 13 or 14 Gy, depending on the antero-posterior diameter of the patient's chest and could, in theory, reduce the efficacy of the treatment. But it is still a reasonable dose, and most of the tumour that is causing symptoms is usually to one side of this midline strip and will still receive the full dose.

Results

It seems from the studies that have been carried out that 60–80% of patients will have an improvement in the major symptoms (cough, haemoptysis and chest pain). Dyspnoea is less well palliated because of the problems of underlying lung disease and persistent lung collapse and consolidation. This palliation seems to last on average for 50% of the patient's remaining life.

Re-Treatment

One problem that is commonly encountered is that of the patient whose symptoms recur after palliative radiotherapy. If this happens quite soon after treatment and the patient's condition is deteriorating quickly it may only be appropriate to give symptomatic therapy. However, when the patient is still fit, has had a good symptom-free period of a few months and clearly has local recurrent tumour it may be right to consider repeating palliative radiotherapy.

A justifiable concern with re-treatment is about spinal cord tolerance, which, unless the tumour is well localized away from the midline, is likely to be exceeded. This worry is probably more theoretical than real because of the short life expectancy of the patient. Our practice is to explain the problem and to repeat the treatment using smaller fractions (usually 20 Gy in 10 fractions) if the patient consents.

Prognosis

Patients with NSCLC too advanced for surgery or radical radiotherapy generally have a poor prognosis. As discussed above, the presence of metastases, significant weight loss and a poor performance status are all associated with a worse prognosis.

Overall, about 50% of patients will survive six months, about 15 to 20% one year and about 5% two years. Patients with a good performance status, however, may live longer and more than 10% may survive to two years.

BRACHYTHERAPY

For some years there has been interest in palliative treatment using intraluminal brachytherapy, which entails the insertion of radioactive materials down the bronchial tree. A machine, the Microselectron, has recently been developed which allows automated insertion of high activity iridium-192 wires down fine bore tubes, sited in the correct position at bronchoscopy. A dose of 8–10 Gy can be delivered to the surface of the tumour in 15 to 30 minutes.

The advantage of this treatment is that a high-dose can be given locally to symptomatic tumour with great accuracy and without using wide-field radiotherapy with its associated side-effects. The treatment can also be repeated without any concern about the dose to the spinal cord.

The disadvantages are the need for a bronchoscopy and day-case admission, and the fact that, because the dose drops quickly away from the radioactive source, larger tumour masses causing extrinsic compression are not adequately irradiated. There have also been occasional reports of fatal haemoptysis due to erosion through into major blood vessels when repeated high-doses have been given, probably because of late radiation necrosis.

The value of this technique compared to conventional large-fraction external beam radiotherapy in terms of efficacy, morbidity and convenience for the patient has not yet been properly evaluated.

CHEMOTHERAPY

Unfortunately, NSCLC is among the more chemoresistant tumours. Cytotoxic drugs are generally considered to be active when they produce response rates greater than 20%. Table 5.4 lists the collective experience from several studies where single-agent response rates have been recorded. As can be seen, only cisplatin, ifosfamide and mitomycin C have been tested in large numbers of patients and shown to be active. But of considerable interest are several new agents which seem, from early (Phase II) studies, to be active in this disease. These are the antimetabolites edatrexate and gemcitabine, the taxanes paclitaxel (Taxol) and docetaxel (Taxotere), a vinca alkaloid, vinorelbine (Navelbine), and two derivatives of camptothecin, irinotecin (CPT-11) and topotecan. If the early promise of these drugs is confirmed, the number of active drugs for NSCLC will be significantly increased and there will be scope for developing new combination regimens.

Combination chemotherapy appears to produce higher response rates than are seen with single agents. The most active combinations are those including cisplatin; the widely used combination of cisplatin with a vinca alkaloid (often vindesine) usually

Table 5.4 Single-agent response rates in NSCLC.

Drug	Number of patients	% Response
Cisplatin	568	21
Ifosfamide	420	26
Mitomycin C	115	20
Vindesine	449	18
Doxorubicin	261	13
Carboplatin	491	11
Etoposide	278	9

gives response rates of between 30 and 35%. Many combinations employing three or more cytotoxic agents have been reported. Three of the most frequently employed regimens have been CAP (cyclophosphamide, doxorubicin and cisplatin), MIC (mitomycin C, ifosfamide and cisplatin) and MVP (mitomycin C, vinblastine and cisplatin). These studies report response rates up to 50%.

Several trials have compared three drugs with combinations including two agents and none has shown any survival advantage for the three-drug regimens. Paradoxically, several trials have shown superior response rates for the two drug regimens, probably resulting from the higher dose intensity which could be achieved when the less myelosuppressive two drug combinations were given.

Although good response rates can be achieved with chemotherapy, this is often at the expense of considerable toxicity and inconvenience to the patient. Whether this translates into an overall benefit for the patient is more difficult to assess and is discussed below.

Adjuvant Chemotherapy

Several studies have investigated the use of chemotherapy following surgery for patients with Stages I – III NSCLC. The aim, as with all adjuvant treatment, is to eradicate any small amount of residual tumour, either local or metastatic, following the well-established oncological principle that cytotoxic agents are more effective when the tumour burden is low.

Only a small number of trials have employed combination chemotherapy and all have included cisplatin, two in combination with doxorubicin and cyclophosphamide. There appeared to be a survival advantage for chemotherapy-treated patients with Stages II and III disease, though the number of patients included was relatively small, and for stage I patients, no survival benefit was observed.

A recent meta-analysis (overview)[5] of these trials has suggested a small benefit for chemotherapy containing cisplatin, but not for chemotherapy with other agents. Several randomized studies are underway with the aim of including larger numbers of patients and for the moment adjuvant chemotherapy after surgery cannot be considered routine.

Neoadjuvant Chemotherapy

The principle of neoadjuvant chemotherapy is to give the drug treatment before surgery in the hope that this would improve survival by reducing tumour volume before resection, improving resectability and eradicating micrometastases. This has been tried in a variety of different tumours with variable success.

At least seven trials have been carried out giving cisplatin-based combination chemotherapy regimens before surgery for NSCLC. These have all been relatively small (the largest included 58 patients) but encouraging response rates were seen and tumour necrosis was documented during surgery. Overall, approximately 70% of patients achieved greater than 50% tumour volume reduction. Complete surgical resection of tumour was achieved in over 50% of patients included in these studies. Survival rates have varied with median survival ranging from 9 to 22 months. Encouragingly one series reported six-year survival rates of 26%.

Two randomized trials in patients with Stage IIIA disease have also been completed and they both showed significant improvement in survival for the patients treated with chemotherapy and surgery compared to those who had surgery alone.

A larger number of series have combined radiotherapy and chemotherapy before surgery with response rates, pathological evidence of tumour necrosis and survival being almost identical to those series which have given chemotherapy alone.

The concept of neoadjuvant treatment in NSCLC is appealing and the results of these trials are encouraging. The data are not yet sufficient for it to be possible to recommend routine neoadjuvant treatment. Further prospective randomized trials that include a large number of patients, are now essential to answer the important questions of whether pre-operative treatment (either chemotherapy or chemotherapy plus radiotherapy) improves surgical resectability and increases survival and for which groups of patients it is beneficial.

Chemotherapy for Advanced Disease

For patients with locally advanced or metastatic NSCLC for whom surgery and radical radiotherapy are not thought appropriate, chemotherapy may be considered. It is important to remember that once patients are thought to be inoperable, or not suitable for radical radiotherapy, all further treatment is aimed at palliation. The use of currently available chemotherapy may not have much effect on survival and its role in treating advanced disease should therefore be limited to symptomatic patients for whom simpler treatments have been unsuccessful.

In trials which compared single-agent chemotherapy with 'best supportive care', there has been no improvement of survival in the chemotherapy group. The results of randomized trials comparing two-drug combinations with single-agent therapy have only shown an improvement in survival in one study where vindesine was compared with the combination of vindesine and cisplatin. For all trials which included cisplatin as the drug in the single-agent group, no survival benefit has been seen.

The question of whether the use of chemotherapy can actually be justified in patients with advanced NSCLC has been addressed in several randomized trials comparing combination chemotherapy with 'best supportive care', which included palliative radiotherapy. All the seven studies which have randomized either two- or three-drug combination regimens against best supportive care (including palliative radiotherapy) have shown survival benefits for the chemotherapy group, although in only three studies did this reach levels of statistical significance. Median survival was increased by an average of approximately 11 weeks, but several criticisms of these studies have been made, including the fact that all included relatively few patients. However, a recent overview of all these trials has confirmed that there is a modest survival benefit from combination chemotherapy but it is not clear whether patients benefit overall in their 'quality of life'.

A number of trials are currently underway comparing cisplatin combination therapy and some of the newer agents with supportive care; they include assessments of quality of life as well as survival. These trials may help to define the true value of chemotherapy in this situation.

COMBINED MODALITY TREATMENT

The unsatisfactory results of surgery and radical radiotherapy for patients with locally advanced (Stages IIIA and IIIB) NSCLC together with the advent of relatively more effective, cisplatin-based chemotherapy regimens has prompted interest in combining chemotherapy with radiotherapy. The drugs might act as radiosensitizers if given concurrently with radiotherapy or might improve survival by controlling micro-metastatic disease.

Randomized trials comparing radical radiotherapy with a combination of radical radiotherapy and chemotherapy (either before radiotherapy or synchronous) have given conflicting results, some showing significant survival benefit and others not. So, despite the theoretical benefits, combined modality treatment still cannot be considered as a standard and should only be carried out in the context of randomized clinical trials.

KEY POINTS

- Surgery is the treatment of choice for patients with NSCLC.
- Selected patients with localized tumours (T1N0 and T2N0) who are inoperable because they are medically unfit may benefit from radical radiotherapy.
- Patients found to have tumour at the resection margin or unexpected N2 disease should receive post-operative radiotherapy if surgery has otherwise been successful.
- Patients with Pancoast tumours may benefit from a combination of surgery and radical radiotherapy.
- The value of radical radiotherapy for patients with bulky Stage IIIB tumours is uncertain.
- Palliative radiotherapy is effective in relieving the local symptoms of many patients with locally advanced NSCLC and can safely be given in one or two large fractions.
- Combination chemotherapy with regimens including cisplatin may be effective for selected patients with Stage IIIA tumours before surgery and for some patients with advanced disease. The overall benefit is still uncertain and so patients should ideally be treated in clinical trials.

REFERENCES

1. Roswit B., Patnom, M.E., Rapp R. **et al**. (1968) The survival of patients with inoperable lung caner: a large scale randomized study of radiation versus placebo. *Radiology,* **90**, 688–697.
2. MRC Lung Cancer Working Party (1994). Randomized trial of surgical resection with or without post-operative radiotherapy in NSCLC. *Lung Cancer,* **11 (Suppl 1)**, 148.
3. MRC Lung Cancer Working Party (1991). Inoperable NSCLC: a MRC randomised trial of palliative radiotherapy with two fractions or ten fractions. *Br. J. Cancer,* **63**, 265–70
4. MRC Lung Cancer Working Party (1992). A MRC randomised trial of palliative radiotherapy with two fractions or a single fraction in patients with inoperable NSCLC and poor performance status. *Br. J. Cancer,* **65**, 934–41.
5. Non-small Cell Lung Cancer Collaborative Group (1995). Chemotherapy in non-small cell lung cancer: a meta-analysis using updated data on individual patients from 52 randomised clinical trials. *Br. Med. J.,* **311,** 899–909.

FURTHER READING

Turrisi A.T. (1991) Radiotherapy for Non-small cell lung cancer. In *Current Topics in Lung Cancer.* Edited by Bunn P.A. Jr. pp. 25–31. Berlin, Heidelberg, New York: Springer-Verlag.
Bunn P. A. Jr. (1991) The role of systemic chemotherapy in Non-small cell lung cancer. In *Current Topics in Lung Cancer.* Edited by Bunn P.A. Jr. pp. 33–46. Berlin, Heidelberg, New York: Springer-Verlag.
Talbot D.C., Smith I.E. (1994) New Drugs in Lung Cancer. In *New Perspectives in Lung Cancer.* Edited by Thatcher N., Spiro S. pp. 143–160. London: BMJ Publishing Group.
Walling J. (1994) Chemotherapy for advanced non-small cell lung cancer. *Respiratory Medicine,* **88,** 649–657.

6 SURGERY

Although surgery is only possible in a limited number of cases, it offers the only real chance of cure and, for selected groups of patients with non-small cell lung cancer (NSCLC), five-year survival rates of up to 60–80% can be achieved. The role of surgery in the management of small cell lung cancer remains controversial (see Chapter 7) and in this chapter we will only discuss surgery for NSCLC.

PRE-OPERATIVE ASSESSMENT

It is very important to make a careful assessment of the patient's suitability for surgical resection so that 'open and close' thoracotomies, or incomplete resections, with their potential morbidity are avoided and the results of surgery are optimal.

There are three areas to consider in assessing a patient for possible surgery: general medical fitness, respiratory status and possible tumour spread. Old age, by itself, is not a contraindication to surgery, provided the patient is otherwise physically fit.

General Medical Fitness

A general assessment of the patient's past history and current medical problems is essential. Because so many lung cancer patients are current or ex-smokers, they have a high incidence of cardiovascular, cerebrovascular and peripheral vascular disease.

Patients with severe peripheral vascular disease, ischaemic heart disease, previous myocardial infarction or stroke are at greater risk of serious problems during and after surgery. Those with other serious medical or psychiatric problems may also be unsuitable for surgery, and alternative management, such as observation or radiotherapy, should be considered.

Respiratory Status

Pulmonary function tests have been discussed in Chapter 3. It is important to consider the patient's actual exercise capacity as well as the results of formal tests. Smaller and older patients have lower predicted lung volumes than young, fit people and so comparison with the predicted lung volumes, rather than just looking at the absolute lung volume results, is also important.

Tumour Spread

It is essential to make as accurate a pre-operative assessment of tumour spread as possible. Mediastinal invasion or nodal spread, or the presence of systemic metastases all generally preclude successful operation.

The investigations of mediastinal tumour spread and systemic metastases are discussed in Chapter 3 and some of the clinical points raised in Chapter 3 are highlighted in Table 6.1.

Intrathoracic Contraindications to Surgery

The most important intrathoracic contraindications to surgery are the presence of pulmonary metastases, direct mediastinal or extensive chest-wall invasion and mediastinal lymph node involvement. The presence of pulmonary metastases is the only absolute contraindication and limited mediastinal disease or chest-wall invasion may sometimes be resectable.

There are no clinical findings that absolutely confirm inoperability, but the finding of pleural effusion, Horner's syndrome, or recurrent laryngeal nerve palsy are very suggestive. Severe chest-wall pain or the presence of a palpable mass, implies chest-wall invasion and a careful assessment, with CT or MR scan, is needed before proceeding to thoracotomy.

Pulmonary metastases or gross mediastinal lymphadenopathy may be obvious on chest X-ray. An elevated hemi-diaphragm may mean phrenic nerve involvement and therefore mediastinal invasion. Rib erosion usually implies chest-wall invasion but does not always exclude resection.

Table 6.1   Clinical features suggesting metastatic disease

Site of Metastasis	History	Physical Examination	Biochemistry
Anywhere	Weight loss	Weight loss/cachexia	
Bone metastases	Bone pain	Bony tenderness	Raised alkaline phosphatase Hypercalcaemia*
Liver Metastases	Anorexia/vomiting Liver Pain Jaundice	Hepatomegaly Liver tenderness	Raised alkaline phosphatase Abnormal liver function tests
Brain Metastases	Headache Seizure Hemiparesis Personality change	Papilloedema Focal neurological signs	

* may be due to ectopic PTH in squamous carcinoma.

The presence of pleural effusion usually means the patient is inoperable, though sometimes a small effusion may simply be related to distal infection (see below).

The value of CT scanning of the mediastinum is discussed in Chapter 3. Enlarged mediastinal nodes may be seen, but do not necessarily contain tumour, although lymph nodes larger than 2 cm in diameter usually contain tumour. Mediastinoscopy should be carried out if significant mediastinal lymphadenopathy (>1 cm) is seen.

Direct invasion of the mediastinum and chest-wall may be obvious on CT scan and preclude surgery but CT findings are not always reliable and MR scanning may be helpful in this situation. The CT features suggestive of mediastinal invasion are listed in Chapter 3.

The following findings at bronchoscopy usually mean that the patient is inoperable:

- tumour in the trachea, at the carina, within 1cm of the carina or in both bronchial trees.
- splaying or broadening of the carina, implying involvement of sub-carinal lymph nodes.

Some carefully selected patients with tumour within 1cm of the carina can undergo successful resection with a sleeve pneumonectomy and carinoplasty but this procedure carries a 20% operative mortality. It is occasionally possible to resect subcarinal lymphadenopathy.

Mediastinoscopy

Mediastinoscopy is an important procedure in the pre-operative assessment because it allows direct inspection and biopsy of the upper mediastinal lymph nodes. It should be carried out if there is any evidence of significant (greater than 1 cm diameter) mediastinal lymphadenopathy on the CT scan. Because size is an unreliable indicator of mediastinal lymph node involvement, in some centres it is routinely done in all patients as part of the staging process.

Mediastinoscopy is a relatively simple procedure performed under general anaesthesia. A small incision is made in the suprasternal notch allowing the mediastinoscope to be passed down behind the sternum. The paratracheal, superior and inferior tracheal lymph nodes can then be seen and felt, and representative samples biopsied. Digital exploration gives an indication of the mobility of the trachea, main bronchus and hilum.

The anterior mediastinal lymph nodes lie in front of the aortic arch and are only accessible by left anterior mediastinotomy. This is sometimes needed in the staging of left upper lobe tumours because these tumours tend to drain to the anterior mediastinal nodes.

Thoracoscopy

Thoracoscopy is not usually needed in routine staging but may be helpful in the rare situation when resection is being considered in a patient with a pleural effusion. If the effusion can be aspirated to dryness, there is no evidence of malignant cells in the aspirate, and the patient is otherwise considered to be operable, thoracoscopy should be carried out. If the formal pleural examination and pleural biopsy both reveal no tumour then it is reasonable to consider the patient for thoracotomy.

Thoracoscopy is also useful in the diagnosis and assessment of patients with malignant mesothelioma (see Chapter 14).

Operative staging

It is important that the tumour is properly staged at the time of surgery for two reasons. Firstly, it may influence the decision on post-operative treatment, such as radiotherapy. Secondly, because the presence and extent of nodal involvement are such strong prognostic indicators, it is essential for any meaningful comparative analysis of survival and outcome.

Full nodal mapping of the mediastinum requires a commitment of time and enthusiasm on the part of the surgeon and pathologist but should be part of the routine surgical management.

The tumour staging system of the American Joint Commission on cancer staging (see Chapter 5) has recently been modified. In particular, T3 now includes tumours that have invaded locally but that may still be surgically resectable. T4 now relates to tumours beyond the limits of conventional surgery. N1 disease continues to apply to peri-bronchial, lobar and hilar nodes on the side of the tumour, whereas N2 disease now indicates ipsilateral mediastinal nodes that might be resectable with curative intent. N3 designates lymphatic spread to sites that cannot be cured by surgery.

SURGICAL TECHNIQUES

The amount of lung that is removed at thoracotomy is determined by the site of the tumour and the extent of lymphatic spread. The traditional operations are lobectomy, right bilobectomy and pneumonectomy.

Lobectomy is the operation of choice for most patients, provided an adequate proximal tumour-free margin (at least 2 cm) can be obtained.

Pneumonectomy is required when the tumour extends into a main bronchus or an adequate margin cannot be achieved by lobectomy alone. Extra-pericardial pneumonectomy is the usual procedure, but intra-pericardial pneumonectomy is needed when the tumour extends along the pulmonary vein or artery or onto the pericardium or phrenic nerve. This more invasive procedure adds to the morbidity and mortality of the operation.

In recent years there has been a trend towards preserving as much viable lung as possible while ensuring adequate clearance of tumour at the resection margin. For this reason, when technically feasible **limited wedge resection** is now undertaken for small, more peripheral tumours, particularly in patients with relatively poor respiratory reserve. However, there is evidence that the local recurrence rate is higher than after lobectomy and, if there is any question about the adequacy of the resection margins, post-operative radiotherapy should be considered.

It is possible that **anatomical segmentectomy,** when feasible, may be as good a cancer operation as traditional methods.

Sleeve resection may be appropriate for some patients with upper lobe tumours that just extend into the intermediate or main bronchi. This operation entails resection of the upper lobe and bronchus together with a short segment of the main bronchus and anastomosis of the main bronchus to the intermediate or left lower lobe bronchus. The re-implanted lobe functions normally and contributes significantly to pulmonary function. This operation is usually reserved for patients with reduced respiratory reserve and has a higher morbidity and mortality as a result.

A few patients with T3N0 tumours invading the chest-wall can be considered for *en bloc* **chest-wall resection** and reconstruction. The morbidity and mortality of this operation is greater than after standard surgery, and the five-year survival is substantially less (20% compared to 60% for successful lobectomies). Few patients will survive five years after an incomplete resection, and so the patients need to be selected very carefully.

Some patients with **Pancoast tumours** may also be suitable for *en bloc* resection, but the extent of local involvement of ribs and brachial plexus by the time a diagnosis is made often precludes this approach. It is usual, though not of proven benefit, to give pre-operative radiotherapy to a dose of 40 Gy followed by post-operative boost to 60 Gy.

Thoracoscopic resection has no major role in the routine management of lung cancer at present though minimally invasive ('keyhole') thoracic surgery is currently being evaluated in a few centres in the United Kingdom.

COMPLICATIONS

As with any major surgical procedure, surgery for lung cancer is not without its complications. These are more frequent after pneumonectomy than after lobectomy or wedge resection but the overall morbidity of surgery is low if patients are selected appropriately.

The complications may be divided into 'early' and 'late' as discussed below.

Early Complications

The patient may have difficulty breathing and coughing because of chest-wall pain following thoracotomy; this can result in **retained secretions** and chest infection.

Adequate post-operative analgesia and physiotherapy are therefore essential and the patients must be nursed in a high dependency area. Patient-controlled analgesia and epidural anaesthesia can be very effective in controlling pain. It is sometimes necessary to perform a mini-tracheostomy to allow adequate suction. Antibiotics, such as a broad-spectrum cephalosporin, are routinely given post-operatively as prophylaxis.

Cardiac dysrhythmias, particularly atrial fibrillation, can occur in the post-operative period, especially after intra-pericardial pneumonectomy and need to be treated appropriately. Sometimes digoxin or beta-blockers are used prophylactically.

Pulmonary thromboembolism can occur, as after any major operation, and prophylactic sub-cutaneous heparin is given peri-operatively. This may, however, preclude epidural anaesthesia.

Systemic hypotension can result from haemorrhage, dysrhythmias or pulmonary thromboembolism and may lead to renal failure, myocardial infarction or stroke.

All patients have an intercostal drain inserted at thoracotomy. After lobectomy or wedge resection, a persistent **pneumothorax** and air leak are not uncommon, but usually resolve with prolonged chest drainage. Re-exploration is rarely needed.

Pulmonary oedema can occur after pneumonectomy when the whole cardiac output is suddenly passing through the single remaining lung. In its severe form it carries a high mortality, but mild to moderate pulmonary oedema is common and responds well to diuretics.

Bronchopleural fistula is a serious complication and is more common following a pneumonectomy than after a partial lung resection. The bronchial wall does not heal well, but following the introduction of stapling methods for bronchial closure, the incidence of fistula formation has been reduced dramatically.

The patient typically develops a slight fever and perhaps minor haemoptysis, and within 24 hours is coughing up pleural fluid. When a fistula develops, immediate action is needed to obtain eventual healing. Bronchoscopy will show the site and size of the fistula. Inserting an intercostal tube to drain the pleura may be all that is necessary for a small fistula, but sometimes surgery is required. An empyema invariably develops and can cause prolonged problems (see below). Other procedures such as sodium hydroxide cautery, omentoplasty, myoplasty or even thoracoplasty are sometimes carried out to seal the fistula.

Empyema can develop with or without a broncho-pleural fistula. Prolonged chest drainage may result in resolution, but occasionally it is impossible to sterilize the pleural space, and rib resection with open drainage is required. This, however, can result in chronic debility and is avoided if possible.

Late Complications

If the lung resection compromises the patient's ventilatory capacity, **respiratory failure** can result. This can also be precipitated by other cardio-respiratory problems such as pneumonia or heart failure and may be accelerated by continued smoking.

Infection of the pleural space may develop late and result in prolonged problems with empyema.

Post-thoracotomy chest pain can be a very troublesome and unpleasant problem. Anaesthesia in the course of the intercostal nerves that are damaged or severed at the time of surgery is inevitable, but some patients go on to develop a dysaesthetic pain in the same area. As with all neuralgic pain, treatment is difficult and often unsatisfactory but benefit can sometimes be gained from tricyclic antidepressants, anticonvulsants or transcutaneous electrical nerve stimulation. Occasionally, nerve blocking or destructive procedures are necessary.

There is some evidence that early intervention with adequate local anaesthesia, especially thoracic epidural, at the time of surgery may prevent this problem.

Depression can occur following thoracotomy as with any major surgery. This can be made worse by chronic disability from a discharging empyema or post-thoracotomy pain. Some patients also fail to come to terms adequately with the fact that they have cancer or that it may recur. Awareness of this potential problem, sensitive enquiry and appropriate therapy are all needed (see Chapter 12).

MORTALITY

In experienced centres, the operative mortality from lobectomy is under 5% and from pneumonectomy is under 10%. Right-sided lobectomy carries a greater risk than left-sided. The higher operative mortality from pneumonectomy is not only because it is a bigger operation but also because those patients needing a pneumonectomy usually have larger tumours. For the same reasons the mortality for intra-pericardial pneumonectomy is higher than extra-pericardial pneumonectomy.

SURVIVAL

The post-operative five-year survival depends on the stage of the tumour; this underscores the importance of careful pre- and intra-operative staging. Stage I tumours (T1 and T2, NO, MO) have a 60% five-year survival and Stage II tumours (T1 and T2, N1 or T3, NO) about a 40% five-year survival.

More advanced tumours, especially those with mediastinal nodal (N2) spread, have significantly poorer five-year survival (IIIA around 20%, IIIB around 5%). The common cause of death following tumour resection remains recurrent tumour (either local or metastatic).

The roles of pre-operative, 'neo-adjuvant' chemotherapy and post-operative chemotherapy and radiotherapy are discussed in Chapter 5.

KEY POINTS

- Pre-operative assessment involves assessing the patient's medical fitness as well as the extent of tumour spread.
- CT scanning of the chest and upper abdomen is an essential part of the pre-operative assessment.
- Mediastinoscopy is the best way of assessing the extent of mediastinal nodal spread.
- The choice of operation depends on the local extent of the tumour and the patient's lung function.
- Selected patients with mediastinal spread may be suitable for radical surgery.
- Operative staging is important for determining prognosis and the need for post-operative radiotherapy.

FURTHER READING

Shields T.W. (1989) Chapter 76: Carcinoma of the Lung. In *General Thoracic Surgery*. Ed. Shields T.W. pp. 890–934. Philadelphia: Lea and Feiberger.

Vincent R.G., Takita H., Lane W.W. *et al.* (1976) Surgical therapy of lung cancer. *J. Cardiovasc. Surg.*, **71**, 581–591.

7 SMALL CELL LUNG CANCER

Small cell lung cancer (SCLC) has one of the highest rates of tumour cell proliferation of all types of malignancy and the clinical course is correspondingly aggressive. Untreated, the median survival from diagnosis is only 5 to 12 weeks depending on the stage at diagnosis. Enormous interest has focused on its treatment because it is among the most responsive tumours to chemotherapy and radiotherapy but, frustratingly, although most patients will benefit from treatment with an improvement in symptoms and increased survival, the tumour usually recurs and ultimately proves fatal. It clearly offers a tantalizing challenge for the development of new treatment strategies.

CLINICAL FEATURES

There are no characteristic clinical features to distinguish SCLC from other primary lung tumours. The primary site is usually in the central bronchial tree and so cough, haemoptysis, dyspnoea and wheeze are all common symptoms. Chest pain can occur, especially if there is mediastinal invasion which can also cause recurrent laryngeal nerve palsy and dysphagia. Spread to mediastinal lymph nodes is common and may lead to superior vena caval obstruction.

When planning treatment for SCLC, it is essential to appreciate that at the time of diagnosis, no matter how small the primary may appear, the disease has almost always metastasized. Autopsy studies have shown the presence of metastases in distant organs in 96% of patients and in one series of patients who had undergone surgical resections of the primary tumour and died from non-cancer causes, 70% of patients had metastases at post-mortem.

A 55-year-old woman presented with haemoptysis. A chest X-ray (Plate 7.1a) showed a right lower zone opacity and right hilar enlargement. Bronchoscopy revealed a tumour in the right lower lobe bronchus, biopsies of which showed small cell carcinoma.

The patient appeared to have limited disease and was in the 'good prognosis' category. She received four courses of combination chemotherapy with cyclophosphamide, doxorubicin, vincristine and etoposide and achieved a complete response (Plate 7.1b). She then had consolidation radiotherapy to the chest.

She remained well and symptom-free for sixteen months, but then developed headaches and a personality change. A CT scan confirmed that she had cerebral metastases and, although she was treated with corticosteroids and cranial radiotherapy, she continued to deteriorate. She died a few months later.

79

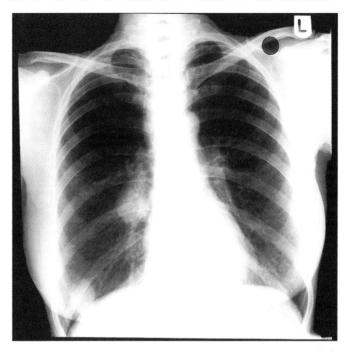

Plate 7.1a   Chest X-ray of a patient with small cell lung cancer in the right lower lobe with right hilar lymphadenopathy.

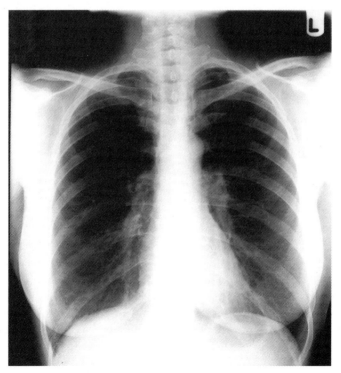

Plate 7.1b   After combination chemotherapy there has been complete response of the tumour and the chest X-ray is normal.

The most frequent sites of metastases are liver, bone, bone marrow and the central nervous system. Abdominal discomfort and biliary obstruction may result from pancreatic or coeliac axis node involvement, and flank pain from adrenal metastases. At presentation, however, most patients will have no symptoms or only minimal discomfort as a result of metastases.

As discussed in Chapters 9 and 11, some paraneoplastic syndromes, especially inappropriate anti-diuretic hormone (ADH) secretion, Cushing's syndrome and the Eaton — Lambert syndrome are all particularly associated with SCLC.

STAGING

The accurate determination of the anatomical extent or stage of disease in patients with SCLC is less important than for NSCLC. Nevertheless, a few, relatively simple investigations help to give an estimate of the amount of tumour, to decide which chemotherapy regimen to use and to allow a comparison of the results of trials using different treatment regimens.

The traditional TNM staging system (see Chapter 5) is inappropriate for SCLC as the tumour is almost always systemic at the time of diagnosis. The Veterans' Administration Lung Cancer Study Group designed a two-stage system for SCLC, dividing patients into those with 'limited' (approximately 30% of patients) and those with 'extensive' disease. 'Limited' disease describes tumour that appears to be confined to one hemithorax (including pleural effusion), mediastinum and ipsilateral supraclavicular lymph nodes. It was originally defined as a tumour volume which could be incorporated into a single 'tolerable' radiotherapy field. 'Extensive' disease is defined as the presence of tumour beyond these sites.

Staging procedures should be chosen for their ability to detect overt metastases quickly and with the least discomfort to the patient because it is important not to delay the start of treatment and the results of extensive staging investigations rarely alter the management. A chest X-ray usually provides enough information to determine whether the intra-thoracic disease is of 'limited' extent and to monitor the response to treatment. CT scanning of the chest may be helpful if the patient is likely to have consolidation radiotherapy (see below).

Our policy is to limit staging investigations to a plain chest X-ray, full blood count with a differential and a full biochemical screen, including serum LDH. Further investigations such as bone scan, liver ultrasound and CT scan of brain, are carried out only if these baseline investigations are abnormal or if clinical symptoms or signs suggest metastases at these sites.

More extensive staging investigations may be appropriate in some clinical trials. Bone marrow biopsies are histologically positive in 10–50% of patients and when staining with monoclonal antibodies is done, involvement may be detected in up to 80% of patients. Up to 50% of patients may also be shown to have liver involvement by scanning or ultrasound at the time of diagnosis, and if CT scans of the abdomen are performed, metastases in the pancreas and adrenal glands may occasionally be demonstrated. CT brain scans may show the presence of metastases in 5% of asymptomatic patients. However the additional information gained from these tests is unlikely to influence the treatment plan for the patient and so they are not routinely performed.

PROGNOSTIC FACTORS

The simple division of patients into those with 'limited' and 'extensive' disease is of considerable value in determining prognosis for patients with SCLC. It has, however, long been realized that within the group who have 'limited' disease, some patients have a poor response to treatment and short survival, whereas a small proportion of patients with 'extensive' disease may be long-term survivors. In an attempt to predict outcome more accurately, a variety of prognostic factors have been examined in multivariate analyses. These have not only allowed a more accurate forecast of the chance of survival for individuals but also enabled some patients to be selected for more aggressive and complex cytotoxic regimens, which for others would simply inflict unnecessary toxicity without providing a significant survival benefit (see below).

Most analyses have shown pre-treatment Performance Status (PS), measured by a variety of scales, to be one of the most important prognostic variables along with disease extent. Other factors found to predict outcome include simple biochemical measurements such as LDH, serum sodium, albumin, and alkaline phosphatase. When planning new randomized studies of treatment, at least some of these factors should be used for stratification.

One prognostic scale that we routinely use to predict outcome is shown in Table 7.1. We would recommend that this or a similar scale is used for choosing patients for particular treatments.

Table 7.1   Adverse prognostic factors in SCLC

Serum Sodium <132 mmol/L
Weight loss >10%
WHO PS >2
Serum bicarbonate <24 mmol/L
Extensive disease (outside one hemithorax and ipsilateral supraclavicular fossa nodes)
Alkaline phosphatase >1.5 × upper limit of normal
LDH >1.5 × upper limit of normal

Patients with none or one of the above classed as 'Good Prognosis'
Patients with two or more as 'Poor Prognosis'

CHEMOTHERAPY

Considerable impetus for the use of chemotherapy in the treatment of SCLC was provided from the results of a placebo-controlled study published in 1969 by the Veterans' Administration Lung Cancer Study Group. This showed a doubling of the median survival for patients given single-agent cyclophosphamide; several subsequent studies comparing radiotherapy alone with radiotherapy and chemotherapy showed significant improvements in survival for the patients given chemotherapy.

Phase II studies have shown that a large number of cytotoxic drugs are active against SCLC. Some of the most frequently used drugs and their single-agent response rates are listed in Table 7.2. Although single-agent therapy produces useful palliation of symptoms and an improvement in median survival to approximately six months, complete remissions and long-term survival are extremely rare.

Table 7.2 Single Agent Response Rates in SCLC

Drug	Response Rate
Carboplatin	58%
Ifosfamide	54%
Etoposide	54%
Vincristine	49%
Doxorubicin	35%
Cyclophosphamide	32%
Methotrexate	30%
CCNU	18%

Combination Chemotherapy

The use of combination chemotherapy in SCLC has improved survival by four- or five-fold compared with untreated patients. Most trials of a variety of different drug combinations in patients with limited disease report overall response rates of 80–90% (50–60% complete) and median survival figures of 12–14 months with two-year survival rates of up to 25%. For patients with extensive stage disease, the overall response rates are slightly lower at about 70% (15–25% complete), the median survival is around 8 months and survival to two years is very rare.

Historical data suggest that combination chemotherapy gives better results than single agents, but surprisingly few trials have prospectively compared the two. Those which have been done suggest that the combination regimens are better in terms of response rate and survival. As more cytotoxic agents are added to combinations, however, the risk of toxicity increases with greater morbidity and mortality.

Attempts have therefore been made to find the optimum number of drugs that will produce an increase in response rate and survival without being associated with unacceptable added toxicity. Comparisons of two-drug with three- and four-drug regimens have been carried out; there seems to be an increase in response rate and survival with increasing numbers of drugs, but there is no evidence that the use of more than four drugs gives any added benefits.

Some of the most commonly used regimens combine cyclophosphamide, doxorubicin and vincristine with or without etoposide (see Table 7.3). Ifosfamide is sometimes substituted for cyclophosphamide because of its lower potential for producing myelosuppression and increased activity. Recently, carboplatin, an analogue of cisplatin, has become available and has one of the highest single-agent response rates seen in SCLC. The combination of ifosfamide, carboplatin, etoposide and vincristine has been given to patients with 'favourable' prognosis SCLC and produced among the best survival figures with up to 32% of patients alive and disease-free two years after treatment. This regimen is, however, profoundly myelo-suppressive and carries significant morbidity and approximately 5% treatment-related mortality.

Table 7.3   Commonly used regimens for SCLC

CAV

Cyclophosphamide	$1,000 \text{ mg/m}^2$ IV day 1
Doxorubicin	45 mg/m^2 IV day 1
Vincristine	1.4 mg/m^2 IV day 1 (max. 2 mg)
Repeated every 21 days	

CAVE

Cyclophosphamide	750 mg/m^2 IV day 1
Doxorubicin	40 mg/m^2 IV day 1
Vincristine	1.4 mg/m^2 IV day 1 (max. 2 mg)
Etoposide	75 mg/m^2 IV day 1
Etoposide	75 mg/m^2 IV or 150 mg/m^2 orally days 2 and 3
Repeated every 21 days	

VICE

Ifosfamide	$5,000 \text{ mg/m}^2$ IV day 1 (with Mesna)
Carboplatin	300 mg/m^2 IV day 1
Etoposide	120 mg/m^2 IV days 1 and 2
Etoposide	240 mg/m^2 orally day 3
Vincristine	1.4 mg/m^2 IV day 8 (max. 2 mg)
Repeated every 21 or 28 days according to FBC	

EP

Etoposide	100 mg/m^2 IV days 1, 2 and 3
Cisplatin	25 mg/m^2 IV days 1, 2 and 3
	or 75 mg/m^2 IV day 1
Repeated every 21 days	

Duration of Chemotherapy

Several trials have investigated the problem of how long chemotherapy should continue, but it is difficult to draw definite conclusions from any of them. The majority of trials suffer from uncontrolled treatments being given at the time of relapse or poor stratification for important prognostic factors. It seems clear, however, that maintenance chemotherapy over many months after the induction of remission confers no survival advantage. The optimum number of courses of chemotherapy seems to be four to six and treatment should be stopped or changed during this period if there is any evidence that the tumour is progressing.

Dose Intensification

There is a considerable amount of data from *in vitro* and animal studies to suggest that for responsive tumours such as SCLC, there is a dose response relationship to chemotherapy, so that the more intensive the chemotherapy (in dose, frequency or both) the greater the effect. In all randomized trials investigating this in patients with SCLC, response rates are better with higher doses and, in at least two trials, survival has been longer. However, the higher-dose regimens caused more toxicity and hospital admissions. These regimens should therefore only be used as part of clinical trials.

Another approach has been to use very high-dose chemotherapy, usually with autologous bone marrow rescue, given after standard treatment has reduced the tumour burden. This strategy is analogous to that now routinely employed in other responsive malignancies (such as acute leukaemia) when patients with a high risk of relapse are identified. The results of several trials have been reported which used such 'late intensification' with a variety of different conditioning regimens and different groups of patients including, in several studies, those who had extensive stage disease at presentation. None has convincingly demonstrated any benefit from this approach.

The treatment-related mortality in these trials was a minimum of 15% and in one trial reached 30%. Despite these apparently negative results, a carefully controlled study using high-dose late intensification in a highly selected group of patients, could still be justified.

Tailoring Chemotherapy to Patient Groups

It is important to select a treatment policy appropriate to each patient. Patients with a good performance status will generally be able to tolerate the toxicity of more intensive chemotherapy regimens and have a better chance of long-term survival. Regimens frequently used in this group of patients often include ifosfamide and carboplatin. The aim is to achieve long-term survival in 10–30% of patients, accepting that significant toxicity and the risk of treatment-related mortality are inevitable.

For the patients, who have a less favourable prognosis (often those with extensive stage disease and other adverse features), regimens including cisplatin and etoposide (PE) or cyclophosphamide, doxorubicin, vincristine with or without etoposide (CAV[E]) are often used.

Unfortunately, patients with SCLC are frequently elderly or have intercurrent illnesses which reduce their ability to tolerate the toxicity of some regimens. For these patients and those with a poor performance status, a regimen of daily oral etoposide has increasingly been employed. A five-day schedule, used in a study involving elderly patients, produced an overall response rate of 79% with 17% complete remissions. Other studies have used more protracted administration with lower doses of etoposide and shown very encouraging response rates with minimal toxicity.

There are a few patients who, for one reason or another, will be unable to tolerate any form of chemotherapy. They should be managed with palliative radiotherapy and other symptomatic measures.

These policies are summarized in Figure 7.1.

RADIOTHERAPY

SCLC is a highly radio-responsive tumour. Although the role of radiotherapy is very much secondary to chemotherapy in the overall management of patients, it is still important.

Consolidation Radiotherapy

For patients with limited-stage disease who have achieved a complete clinical response to chemotherapy, it is usual to give a course of radiotherapy to the mediastinum and site of primary disease. The available evidence suggests that this policy of 'consolidation' reduces the risk of local relapse but does not affect overall survival which is more determined by systemic relapse. We feel that once a patient has undergone chemotherapy and has completely responded, it is important to maximize the chances of controlling the local disease in the chest, and we therefore usually recommend consolidation radiotherapy.

Outside the constraints of clinical trials, when it may be very important to establish the completeness of clinical response, we do not usually confirm the X-ray appearance of complete response by repeating a bronchoscopy. There are, however, a number of patients who respond well to chemotherapy but whose X-rays never completely return to normal. Provided there is no obvious mass visible and the remaining abnormality is consistent with post-inflammatory scarring, our policy is to treat these patients as if they are in complete remission.

Patients who do not achieve a complete clinical response and are asymptomatic are probably best left alone to enjoy their period of remission. They are likely to relapse in due course and radiotherapy can be kept in reserve to treat them palliatively

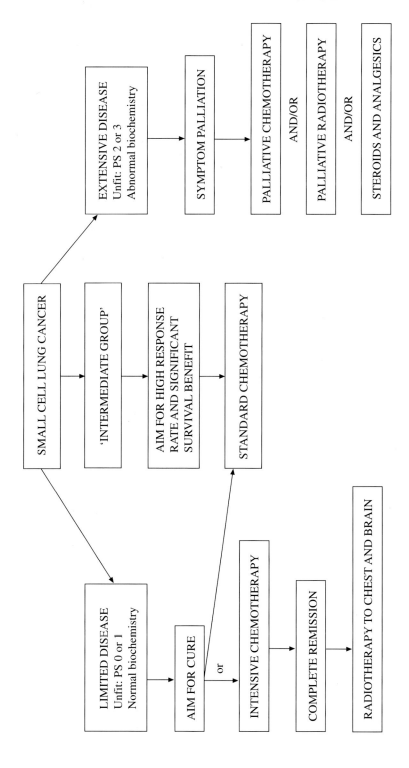

Figure 7.1 Management policies for SCLC

when they do. Also, there is no point in giving consolidation radiotherapy to patients with extensive disease at presentation even if they achieve a complete remission with chemotherapy because they are as likely to relapse outside the chest as
within.

When planning consolidation radiotherapy, the conventional view is that it is important to try to cover the whole area that was originally involved by tumour as shown
on a chest X-ray before chemotherapy. This is a counsel of perfection and in reality
may not always be possible to achieve for two reasons.

Firstly, there is often collapse and consolidation associated with the tumour which
may obscure its actual extent and it is often inappropriate to include the whole area
of consolidation in the treatment volume. A CT scan may give more information,
but even on CT it is often difficult to distinguish inflammatory change from tumour.
Secondly, the tumour at presentation may have been so big or, occasionally, so
peripheral that an unacceptably large volume of normal lung would have to be
included. In both these cases some compromise and arbitrary decisions may have to
be made about the appropriate volume to treat. Reassuringly, recent research has
suggested that adequate treatment to the presumed site of origin of the primary and
the adjacent mediastinum may give as good results as treatment to the whole 'pre-
chemotherapy' volume.

The most appropriate dose of consolidation radiotherapy is also controversial.
Our policy is to give 40 Gy midplane in 15 fractions over three weeks by parallel
opposed fields. This dose is radiobiologically equivalent in terms of acute effects
(and probably tumour-cell kill) to 50 Gy in 25 fractions, but, because of the large
fractions has a greater risk of giving late toxicity (although whether this is clinically
relevant is debatable). It is higher than the tolerance of the spinal cord and the
spine must be shielded from the posterior field for the final three to five fractions,
trying to keep the cord dose below 35 Gy. This has the theoretical disadvantage of
reducing the dose to the mediastinum in the midline, but there is no good evidence
that this is a problem. An alternative, more complex, but more satisfactory technique
is to use a posterior oblique field for the last few fractions. It can be argued that
ideally patients should have CT planned, multifield radical treatment giving at least
50 Gy in 2 Gy fractions in this situation, but, in the absence of convincing evidence of
a survival advantage, we do not feel that this use of limited resources is appropriate.

Consolidation radiotherapy is usually well tolerated. Nausea and anorexia
sometimes occur but vomiting is unusual. The greatest problem is often radiation
oesophagitis (see Chapter 5) which can be worse in patients who have had
anthracyclines as part of their initial chemotherapy. It usually resolves within one or
two weeks of finishing radiotherapy but can sometimes be persistently troublesome.

Radiation pneumonitis (see Chapter 5) may also give transient symptoms of cough
and dyspnoea at six to eight weeks after radiotherapy and, after six months, there is
almost always chest X-ray evidence of fibrosis, well demarcated within the area irradiated. If the volume of lung irradiated has been appropriately planned it is unlikely
that the fibrosis will cause clinical symptoms. In fact, an advantage of using parallel
opposed fields rather than a three-field plan is that the volume of normal lung irradiated is usually less.

Over recent years there has been considerable research interest in giving radio-therapy in combination with the initial chemotherapy to fit patients who have limited disease. There are some theoretical advantages to this approach — the chance of resistant tumour cells developing and the overall length of the primary treatment are reduced — and some evidence to suggest that there is a survival advantage. However, there is also an increased risk of serious toxicity and so this approach should, for the moment, be regarded as experimental and should only be used in the context of clinical trials.

Prophylactic Cranial Irradiation

For patients who achieve a complete remission after chemotherapy there is a 20% risk of subsequently developing brain metastases. Although for many patients this occurs at the same time as, or shortly after other systemic or local relapse, for some this will be the first and only site of relapse. There is some evidence that the intact blood brain barrier prevents access of most cytotoxic drugs to the brain and so micro-metastases in the brain might not be adequately treated by systemic chemotherapy.

This problem has led to the policy of giving prophylactic cranial irradiation (PCI) to selected patients, usually those with limited disease who achieve a complete remission with induction chemotherapy. The available evidence suggests that this reduces the risk of brain metastases to about 8% but does not affect overall survival. A dose of 24–30 Gy over 10–15 fractions is given to the whole brain.

PCI is associated with some acute side-effects. Patients often feel tired and may develop a mild headache. Nausea and anorexia are common but vomiting is unusual. An acute erythematous reaction in the skin of the scalp will occcur after 3 weeks and this may progress to dry desquamation, particularly if they have previously received anthracyclines. Patients need to be warned that recovery of alopecia will be delayed and may be incomplete.

Over the past few years, however, a number of patients who have had PCI and have survived for more than two years have developed a syndrome of ataxia and memory failure suggestive of diffuse cerebral damage. The actual incidence of this problem seems to vary considerably between different series and, because there are so many variables in terms of the dose of PCI, the cytotoxic drugs given, and, perhaps most critically, the timing of PCI in relation to the chemotherapy, it is difficult to know exactly what the causative factors are. The dose given is not normally considered to cause late brain damage and the drugs are not usually neurotoxic, and so there must be some combination or time relation of the radiotherapy with chemotherapy that is potentially damaging.

In the light of this, it would be wrong to give a strong recommendation about the use of PCI. Certainly in our experience, giving PCI (30 Gy in 10 or 15 fractions) after completion of the chemotherapy seems to be relatively safe and we have not seen the severe and frequent problems reported by others. A large randomised trial is in progress in Europe including the United Kingdom, and this will perhaps eventually give us clear guidelines.

Palliative Radiotherapy

Radiotherapy is very useful in the palliation of local symptoms in patients with recurrent and metastatic tumour or in those who are thought to be too frail to tolerate systemic chemotherapy. The prognosis of these patients is necessarily poor and it is usually appropriate to treat them with large single fractions (see Chapter 5).

SURGERY

With the realisation that at the time of diagnosis, SCLC is a systemic disease in the majority of patients, the use of surgery to resect the primary tumour was largely abandoned during the early 1970s. A large MRC study showed radiotherapy to be the better primary treatment of patients with potentially operable SCLC and a subsequent study showed identical survival rates for patients considered operable who either subsequently underwent resection or were managed symptomatically.

A review of previous series published during the 1960s did, however, reveal that, in some reports, five-year survival rates of approximately 10% were achieved. Two series reporting results of treatment of the few patients (about 1%) who present with a solitary nodule showed prolonged survival rates (more than 10 years) in more than a third of patients. Further support for this approach was provided by Meyer[1] who combined adjuvant chemotherapy with surgery for stages I and II tumours and reported 80% survival rates at 30 months. The Veterans Administration Surgical Oncology Group reviewed their experience of patients with SCLC who had undergone potentially curative surgical resection.[2] These patients were randomized to receive post-operative chemotherapy or surgery alone and an overall five-year survival rate of 23% was documented. Post-operative chemotherapy improved survival a little, but there was a group of carefully staged patients with early stage disease who were long-term survivors after surgery alone.

Several groups are now considering surgical resection for the relatively few patients who present with apparently localized pulmonary nodules and are combining this with chemotherapy. The rationale is that complete surgical excision may reduce the rate of local relapse following chemotherapy alone (which in some series approaches 75%).

Patients who have a previously undiagnosed peripheral tumour that turns out, following thoracotomy and complete resection, to be SCLC should probably have two to four courses of post-operative chemotherapy if they are fit enough. Those with a pre-operative pathological diagnosis of SCLC and true stage I disease after staging that includes a mediastinoscopy, may also be considered for resection and post-operative chemotherapy.

The use of preoperative chemotherapy is an alternative approach that is being increasingly considered for patients with stage I disease. A study from Toronto has documented the results of such an approach and, at the time of reporting, the median survival had not been reached. The same research group reported no difference in outcome for patients whose surgery was preceded or followed by chemotherapy. An ongoing American study is attempting to answer the question of whether surgery following complete response to chemotherapy is of value by randomising patients to these two approaches.

TREATMENT OF RELAPSED SCLC

The majority of patients who respond to first-line chemotherapy will ultimately relapse. When this happens, the results of treating them again with chemotherapy are generally poor with response rates of only 20–25% and a median survival from relapse of only three or four months. The chance of a response to second-line chemotherapy is better if the relapse occurs more than one year after initial treatment. At this stage, the disease must be regarded as incurable and so the treatment offered is palliative and the aim is to extend life with good quality. It may be possible to induce a response either using the same drugs as were used initially, or else different drugs to which the tumour may not be resisitant.

Our policy is to treat relapsed patients with palliative radiotherapy if they have local symptoms in an area that can be irradiated (see above). However, if they have widespread disease or systemic symptoms, are reasonably fit and have had a remission of over a year, we would consider treatment with combination chemotherapy as outlined above. If the patient is frailer but chemotherapy is still being considered, then seven to ten days of oral etoposide repeated every three weeks, can be used. Otherwise patients should be treated symptomatically with steroids, opiates etc. (see Chapter 10).

The ultimate cause of treatment failure in SCLC is relapse with chemotherapy-resistant tumour. This may represent overgrowth of inherently resistant tumour cells or else be the result of cells somehow acquiring resistance after exposure to the cytoxic drugs.

There has been considerable laboratory research into drug-resistance in many tumours, including SCLC, and a number of possible mechanisms identified. These include alterations in the detoxification enzyme, glutathione-S-transferase, alterations in the DNA repair enzyme topoisomerase-II, and the development of an abnormal cell membrane protein (p-glycoprotein). This remains an area of active laboratory and clinical research.

KEY POINTS

- Small cell lung cancer is as an aggressive tumour and even at presentation most patients have metastases, often occult.
- Simple assessment of performance status and clinical evidence of metastases give enough information to estimate prognosis and determine appropriate management.
- Combination chemotherapy is the treatment of choice and an increase in survival is possible for most patients, but an attempt at cure is only possible for a selected few.
- Patients with limited disease who achieve a complete response to chemotherapy should be considered for consolidation radiotherapy and cranial irradiation.
- Most patients will eventually relapse. More chemotherapy is then palliative but a useful remission may be possible in more than half of those who relapse after 12 months. Otherwise palliative radiotherapy may be used.
- The role of surgery in small cell lung cancer remains controversial.

REFERENCES

1. Meyer J.A. (1985) Effect of histologically verified TNM stage on disease control in treated small cell lung cancer. *Cancer*, **55**, 1747–1752.
2. Shields T.W., Higgins G.A., Matthews M.J. *et al.* (1982) Surgical resection in the management of small cell carcinoma of the lung. *J. Thorac. Cardiovasc. Surg.*, **84**, 481–488.

FURTHER READING

Hansen H.H. (1993) Chemotherapy of small cell lung cancer. In *Lung Cancer- Frontiers of Science and Treatment*. Edited by Motta G. pp. 557–563. Genoa: Grafica LP.
Ihde D., Pass H. and Glatstein E. (1993) Small cell lung cancer. In *Cancer: Principles and Practice of Oncology*. 4th edn. Edited by De Vita, Hellman and Rosenberg. Philadelphia: J.B. Lippincott and Co.

8 MANAGEMENT OF METASTATIC DISEASE

Metastases are all too frequent in all types of lung cancer either at presentation or in the later stages of the disease. The common sites of clinically obvious metastases are liver, bone, lymph nodes, lung, brain and skin, but metastases can occur anywhere and are often found to be widespread at post-mortem examination. With the advent of routine upper abdominal CT scanning or ultrasound, adrenal metastases are being diagnosed more frequently although they are rarely symptomatic.

Systemic chemotherapy is the logical treatment of widespread disease. Unfortunately, as is described in Chapters 5 and 7, the chemotherapy of NSCLC cannot be yet regarded as standard and the second-line treatment of relapsed patients with SCLC is also unsatisfactory. There are therefore a large number of patients with troublesome symptoms from their metastases which need alternative management.

In this chapter we will briefly describe how to deal with some of the common problems due to metastatic disease.

BONE METASTASES

Bone metastases are a frequent cause of distressing symptoms. They usually present with pain especially in weight-bearing parts of the skeleton such as vertebrae, pelvis and femora. Local tenderness is a useful clinical feature that helps distinguish bone metastases from benign causes of skeletal pain; it is probably due to an associated inflammatory reaction. Bone metastases can also result in pathological bone fracture especially of vertebrae, femur and humerus.

The finding of a raised level of alkaline phosphatase is a useful pointer to bone metastases but is not diagnostic because of the other possible causes such as liver disease, Paget's disease of bone or recent bone injury or surgery.

X-rays of the symptomatic area often show up the metastases, which in lung cancer are almost always lytic. But they can be normal in which case an isotope bone scan which is more sensitive, is usually diagnostic. Bone scans do sometimes need to be interpreted with caution especially if there is a solitary area of increased isotope uptake or a history of trauma or in an elderly patient who may have benign osteoporotic collapse of vertebrae. MRI scanning may clarify the diagnosis.

The pain of bone metastases should be managed first of all with non-steroidal anti-inflammatory drugs (such as naproxen) which can often give significant benefit through their effect on the prostaglandin-mediated inflammation surrounding the metastases. Often though, stronger analgesics such as an opiate are needed (see Chapter 11).

Palliative radiotherapy can be very effective in relieving pain and should be considered in all patients who are not too ill or frail. In most cases a single fraction of 8 or 10 Gy is all that is needed, entailing only one visit to the radiotherapy department. There may be very occasional patients, who appear to have solitary metastases and are otherwise relatively well, for whom a more prolonged course to a higher dose might be justified in order to give longer symptom control or possibly to prevent pathological fracture. Usually, however, when patients with lung cancer have bone metastases their prognosis is poor and such treatment is not appropriate.

Pathological fracture of a long bone such as femur or humerus is usually extremely painful, distressing and disabling. If the patient is fit enough, surgical intervention should be considered. Intra-medullary nails can be put in relatively easily and can restore mobility and reduce the pain quite quickly. Prophylactic pinning of large metastases should also be considered, particularly if there is significant erosion of the bone cortex.

It is not really clear whether or not it is necessary to irradiate bones after they have been pinned and are therefore stable. It is, however, common practice; again, a single fraction is probably all that is needed, using a generous field to cover the site of metastasis but not the whole length of the nail.

Metastases in the base of the skull can produce particular problems with headache and cranial nerve palsies due to entrapment. They may produce confusing clinical signs and be hard to diagnose, particularly as conventional imaging of this area is difficult. MRI may be helpful in this situation. They should be managed with high-dose dexamethasone and palliative radiotherapy .

BRAIN METASTASES

Symptomatic brain metastases occur quite often in patients with lung cancer and sometimes can be the presenting feature of the illness. Up to 20% of patients with SCLC may develop them before death and they are more frequent in patients with adenocarcinoma than with other types of NSCLC.

Brain metastases should be suspected in any patient developing neurological symptoms and signs, especially those of gradual onset and associated with the features of raised intracranial pressure. The clinical picture can, however, be very variable and there may be a sudden onset mimicking a cerebrovascular accident even without overt bleeding into the metastasis. The symptoms and signs of raised intracranial pressure can also be variable and the complete picture of early-morning headache, projectile vomiting and papilloedema is unusual. Other presenting symptoms can be seizures, either generalized or focal, and confusion or personality change.

The diagnosis should be established by CT scanning. Isotope brain scanning is not as reliable and can give false negatives, though, in the absence of a CT scan, a positive isotope scan is diagnostic. If possible, corticosteroids should not be started until the CT scan has confirmed the diagnosis, as the oedema surrounding the metastases may resolve and so make detection more difficult. This is, however, a counsel of perfection because of the distressing symptoms and the delays in getting scans. Patients with fits should be started on adequate doses of anticonvulsants as soon as possible.

As soon as the diagnosis has been confirmed start the patient on high-dose corticosteroids. Dexamethasone 16 mg daily is usually adequate, but care is needed using a dose this high (equivalent to 100 mg of prednisolone) because of the problems of diabetes mellitus, fluid retention, hypertension and oropharyngeal thrush.

If there is a significant improvement in the symptoms, the patient should have radiotherapy to the whole brain. A dose of 20 Gy in five fractions has been shown to be as effective as more prolonged schedules. It is usual to cover the whole brain even if the metastases are well localized because it is very likely that they are multiple and the wide-field radiotherapy does not increase the morbidity significantly at this dose. It is not necessary, however, to take elaborate precautions in planning to include the cribriform plate and the whole of the temporal lobes unless there is a particular clinical indication.

Cranial radiotherapy is usually well tolerated. Mild nausea and headaches sometimes occur, but acute cerebral oedema is unusual, particularly if corticosteroids have been started beforehand. There will, however, be an acute skin reaction with erythema, dry desquamation and hair loss occurring after 10 to 14 days. Patients can be reassured that their hair is likely to regrow over the next few months.

One important reason for giving cranial radiotherapy is to prevent patients from getting the side-effects of prolonged high-dose corticosteroids. As soon as the radiotherapy has started it is usually possible to reduce the steroids. Our policy is to halve the dose every week down to 2 mg daily until the patient is reviewed at about four weeks provided that there is no deterioration in the symptoms.

Patients who do not improve with high-dose steroids are unlikely to improve with radiotherapy. This is probably because if there is no improvement by reducing oedema, there is likely to be substantial structural damage in the brain which will not improve even if the tumour itself shrinks.

Patients with SCLC who have brain metastases at presentation and have therefore not yet had cytotoxic chemotherapy can be treated with drugs and have a good chance of responding. Although the blood brain barrier normally prevents access of most cytotoxic drugs to the brain, it is thought that established metastases break down this barrier allowing the drugs to penetrate.

LIVER METASTASES

Liver metastases are often found incidentally during the initial diagnostic investigation of patients and are usually asymptomatic at that stage. Although they may cause a patient to present with overt jaundice and liver failure, it is more typical for the initial symptoms to be rather vague. General malaise, anorexia, epigastric fullness and a sensation of bloating are common complaints. More severe hepatic pain can occur if there is haemorrhage into a large metastasis of if there is liver capsule distension.

If chemotherapy is not being considered, the patients should be managed symptomatically with corticosteroids (prednisolone 20–30 mg per day), which may improve the systemic symptoms, and analgesics. Palliative radiotherapy (20 Gy in 5 fractions or 30 Gy in 10 fractions, covered with corticosteroids and appropriate antiemetics) may be helpful for occasional patients with severe liver pain or obstructive jaundice due to nodal enlargement at the porta hepatis.

ADRENAL METASTASES

Adrenal metastases are frequently seen at post-mortem but do not often cause clinical symptoms. Occasional patients do however get loin pain as a result and sometimes a mass is palpable. Haematuria can also occur if there is invasion into the kidney. Palliative radiotherapy (20 Gy in 5 fractions) may be helpful.

SKIN METASTASES

Tumour deposits in the skin may be distressing for the patient because they are such an obvious sign of their disease, but they do not often cause severe symptoms. They may, however, be painful or inconvenient and sometimes fungate and bleed. They can be very simply treated with single fractions (10–15 Gy) of electron or orthovoltage radiotherapy .

KEY POINTS

- Metastases are a very common cause of symptoms.
- Bone metastases can be simply treated with palliative radiotherapy.
- Metastases in long bones may need pinning to prevent pathological fracture.
- CT scanning is the investigation of choice for suspected brain metastases.
- Patients with brain metastases should be treated with dexamethasone and, if there is a good symptomatic response, be considered for palliative radiotherapy.
- Palliative radiotherapy may be useful for relieving local symptoms from metastases at most sites.

---

9 PARANEOPLASTIC ENDOCRINE SYNDROMES

Patients with cancer may have a variety of symptoms and signs that are directly related to their primary tumour or to metastases. However, diagnostic problems may arise when patients present with symptoms or signs that are not directly related to local tumour, but are caused by one of a variety of paraneoplastic syndromes. They can become profoundly unwell from the metabolic disturbances associated with cancer and can die without appropriate treatment because the correct diagnosis is missed. It is clearly essential to be aware of these conditions.

HYPERCALCAEMIA

Hypercalcaemia is the commonest tumour-related metabolic disorder and may be life-threatening by the time the patient seeks medical help. It can occur with any type of lung cancer but is most commonly associated with squamous cell tumours.

Symptoms

The symptoms of hypercalcaemia can be varied and their severity may not be related to the serum calcium level. Fatigue, lethargy, constipation, nausea, thirst, polydipsia and polyuria are the commonest early symptoms. At a later stage, severe dehydration, muscle weakness, renal failure and convulsions may occur. Ultimately coma and death will follow if treatment is not started quickly.

Many of these symptoms are often seen in patients with advanced lung cancer without hypercalcaemia, particularly if they are on opiates for pain. But it is important to exclude hypercalcaemia because it is potentially treatable and its correction may significantly improve the patient's well-being.

Pathophysiology

The high serum calcium level results from increased calcium release from bone. The underlying cause was originally thought to be direct bone destruction by the tumour, but it is now clear that it is due to stimulation of osteoclast activity by factors released from the malignant cells. Prostaglandins, 1,25-dihydroxy vitamin D3 and a variety of cytokines including transforming growth factor, interleukin-1, platelet-derived growth factor and tumour necrosis factor may all be released locally by tumour cells in bone metastases and have this effect.

In squamous cell carcinomas, however, the factor responsible is frequently a protein which shares some structural homology with parathyroid hormone and acts in the same way. This may be released in sufficient amounts from the primary tumour or metastatic sites other than bone to have a 'non-metastatic' effect on bone resorption and produce hypercalcaemia. Treatment of the primary tumour may lead to improvement in hypercalcaemia.

Management

Patients with modestly raised serum calcium levels (up to 2.9 mmol/l) who are asymptomatic may need no specific treatment. If it is truly a non-metastatic phenomenon it may respond to treatment of the primary tumour with surgery or radiotherapy.

It is more usual, however, to find patients with moderate to severe symptoms and higher levels of serum calcium, who will need more urgent and intensive treatment.

At least 3 litres of saline should be given quite quickly, because most patients are hypovolaemic. This will often improve their clinical status rapidly and correcting hypovolaemia and total body sodium depletion will also inhibit renal tubular absorption of calcium. Normal saline should be infused at a rate of 300–400 ml per hour for 4–6 hours, but this will depend on the cardiovascular and renal function of the patient. Regular monitoring of electrolyte levels is important, and potassium and magnesium should be replaced as necessary. The addition of a loop diuretic, such as frusemide, increases urinary calcium excretion, but should be avoided during the period of hypovolaemia.

Although fluid replacement is the essential first step in the management of hypercalcaemia, it is unlikely to reduce the serum calcium level by very much and additional treatment to reduce calcium reabsorption is usually needed.

The management of patients with hypercalcaemia has been improved in the past few years with the availability of bisphosphonates which are potent inhibitors of bone resorption. The most frequently used compounds are etidronate, clodronate and pamidronate. Etidronate is available in an oral formulation, but as a result of variable absorption by this route, bisphosphonates are generally given intravenously. The commonly used drugs and dosages are shown in Table 9.1. Approximately 90% of patients become normocalcaemic and this effect lasts a median of three weeks, at which time the treatment can be repeated.

Some other drugs inhibit osteoclast activity. Corticosteroids were often used in the past but are only useful when they have a cytostatic action on the underlying tumour, for instance in lymphoma and multiple myeloma. They do not significantly reduce serum calcium levels in patients with lung cancer.

Table 9.1   Bisphosphonates used for hypercalcaemia

Drug	Dose
Pamidronate	15–60 mg slow IV infusion
Clodronate	1.5 G slow IV infusion
Etidronate	7.5 mg/kg daily for three days, IV infusion
	20 mg/kg *orally* for 30 days

Calcitonin not only inhibits bone resorption but increases renal calcium excretion. It has a rapid onset of action (within four hours) and minimal toxicity. Its value is limited by its failure to produce prolonged control of hypercalcaemia and so it should only be used in the management of acute episodes. Doses of 400 IU every six hours given intramuscularly can be given but use beyond 48 hours is not advised. It may therefore occasionally be useful in cases of severe hypercalcaemia to control the serum calcium level until the effect of bisphosphonates starts.

Other agents which have been used to reduce serum calcium levels are phosphate, prostaglandin inhibitors, sulphate, citrate, gallium nitrate and mithramycin. These all may reduce serum calcium levels but are now rarely used, because of their relative lack of efficacy or their toxicity.

INAPPROPRIATE ADH SECRETION

A number of benign and malignant conditions can produce the syndrome of inappropriate ADH secretion (SIADH), but it is most commonly associated with SCLC. It is caused by secretion from the tumour cells of a polypeptide with ADH-like action on the renal tubules, which results in net water retention.

The clinical presentation is very variable. Often it is only discovered incidentally by finding a low serum sodium level on routine biochemical screening and patients are usually asymptomatic with sodium levels down to 130 mmol/l. Below that level they may complain of tiredness, weakness and lethargy and with levels less than 125 mmol/l they may become increasingly confused and disorientated. Convulsions and coma can occur with levels below about 115 mmol/l. Although there is water retention there is no oedema.

The diagnosis can be confirmed by measuring urinary and plasma osmolality. Normally the serum osmolality is greater than 280 mmol/kg but, in SIADH it can be as low as 190 mmol/kg and the urinary osmolality is inappropriately higher than that of the serum, usually more than 500 mmol/kg.

It is important to exclude other causes of hyponatraemia including diuretic use, cardiac and renal failure, polydipsia and adrenal failure. Cytotoxic agents including cyclophosphamide may also reduce free water excretion and can, rarely, cause hyponatraemia. If the patient is comatose or confused it is also important to exclude other causes of confusion and coma particularly if the serum sodium level is greater than 125 mmol/l.

When a diagnosis of SIADH has been made, the definitive treatment is to treat the tumour with chemotherapy. If the patient is symptomatic or has severe hyponatraemia (less than 130 mmol/litre) restriction of total fluid intake to between 500 ml and 1 litre per day will lead to a slow but steady increase in serum osmolality.

When the serum sodium level is less than 125 mmol/l, or the patient is severely symptomatic, it may be necessary to correct the hyponatraemia before chemotherapy starts, especially if fluid loading is part of the regimen. Demeclocycline, a tetracycline antibiotic, blocks the action of ADH on the renal tubules. It should be given in a dose of 300 mg to 400 mg eight-hourly, with a maintenance dose of 200 mg eight-hourly once the serum sodium level has returned to normal.

If the patient is comatose or having fits, more aggressive treatment may be needed. The excretion of free water can be increased by infusing hypertonic saline with intravenous frusemide. This is a potentially hazardous procedure and requires regular monitoring of serum and urinary electrolytes. It should only be undertaken as a last resort and is very rarely necessary.

CUSHING'S SYNDROME

Abnormal production of ACTH has been demonstrated by radio-immunoassay in the blood and tumour extracts of approximately 40% of all patients with SCLC. This figure is higher than the number of patients observed to have clinical manifestations of Cushing's syndrome — less than 2% of patients with all histological subtypes of lung cancer and up to 5% of patients with SCLC.

Carcinoma of the bronchus is associated with over 50% of all cases of tumour-related Cushing's syndrome, and bronchial carcinoid causes a further 10% of cases (see Chapter 13).

Patients may present with a variety of symptoms and signs. Typically the patient complains of muscle weakness and lethargy, and systemic hypertension, peripheral oedema, hypokalaemia and hyperglycaemia are all common findings. The classic features of Cushing's syndrome such as cutaneous striae, buffalo hump, pigmentation and moon face, however, are not often seen with carcinoma of the bronchus, as the tumour generally progresses before they occur. They may, however, be seen in patients with bronchial carcinoid when the course of the disease is more indolent.

As with all paraneoplastic syndromes, it is important to be aware of the possibility of production of ectopic ACTH in patients with a diagnosis of lung cancer. The presence of lethargy, muscle weakness, weight loss and oedema may all be attributed to non-specific effects of the tumour itself, rather than to Cushing's syndrome. It is important to check the serum biochemistry from time to time and the finding of hypokalaemic alkalosis and hyperglycaemia raise the suspicion of the true cause.

Investigation should include the measurement of 24-hour urinary free cortisol where levels between 100 and 1000 mg/day may occur. There will be loss of the normal ability to suppress serum cortisol levels with dexamethasone when a single 8mg dose of dexamethasone is given at midnight and plasma cortisol levels checked eight hours later. Measurement of the plasma ACTH level can help to confirm the diagnosis with values greater than 200 pg/ml strongly suggestive of ectopic ACTH production. Lower levels do not, however, rule out this diagnosis.

Once the diagnosis of Cushing's syndrome is made, treatment is aimed at reducing the volume of the primary tumour. Surgery for bronchial carcinoid and NSCLC can result in rapid reductions of ACTH levels and resolution of the symptoms. Similar benefits can follow combination chemotherapy for the treatment of SCLC.

Symptomatic measures include the use of metyrapone, aminoglutethimide or mitotane to reduce adrenal corticoid production and these may be helpful if treatment of the primary tumour is unsuccessful.

KEY POINTS

- Hypercalcaemia is the commonest metabolic disorder in patients with lung cancer.
- Hypercalcaemia should be excluded in any patient with thirst, polyuria, constipation or mental confusion.
- Rehydration and bisphosphonates are the mainstay of treatment of hypercalcaemia.
- SIADH is common in patients with SCLC and if the serum sodium level is less than 115 mmol/l, may cause serious problems.
- SIADH should be managed initially with fluid restriction and anti-tumour treatment.
- Demeclocycline (300 mg, t.d.s.) may be needed in cases of severe persistent SIADH.
- Cushing's syndrome is uncommon but may cause hypokalaemia and muscle weakness without the other, more usual clinical signs.

FURTHER READING

Steward W.P. (1991) Metabolic complications of malignancy. *Medicine International*, **92**, 3839–3841.

Bunn Jr. P., Ridgway E.C. (1993) Paraneoplastic Syndromes. In *Cancer: Principles and Practice of Oncology*. 4th edn. Edited by De Vita, Hellman and Rosenberg. Philadelphia: J.B. Lippincott and Co.

10 MANAGEMENT OF ADVANCED SYMPTOMATIC DISEASE

The majority of patients with lung cancer will die of the disease and so it is essential for clinicians to be able to manage the distressing symptoms of advanced recurrent and metastatic tumour skilfully. There is always a difficult balance to be maintained between aggressive intervention and minimal treatment, but it is important to consider the symptoms and problems carefully and to offer the best available management. There is nothing more discouraging for a patient, already burdened with the knowledge that he has a fatal disease, than to feel that his doctors think that there is nothing more that can be done. There are always things that can be done even if it is just the fine adjustment of analgesics or the sorting out of constipation.

In this chapter we will describe some of the common problems of patients with advanced disease and give some suggestions about how best to manage them.

SUPERIOR VENA CAVAL OBSTRUCTION

Superior vena caval obstruction (SVCO) occurs when tumour compresses the superior vena cava (SVC) in its course through the upper mediastinum to the right of the trachea. It can be caused by a medially sited primary tumour in the right upper lobe or, more commonly, by metastatic tumour in right paratracheal lymph nodes.

The clinical features are of progressive neck swelling followed by facial and upper limb oedema. These symptoms are often worse in the morning and improve during the day if the patient is upright and mobile. Dyspnoea is not a feature unless there is associated tracheal compression and stridor. Although the symptoms can get worse quite rapidly to start with, they do tend to stabilize after a few days when chest wall collateral veins have opened up.

The clinical findings are of a patient with a swollen neck and fixed engorgement of the external jugular and superficial arm veins (Plate 2.4). There may be associated facial and hand oedema and there are usually obvious collateral veins over the chest wall. The diagnosis is often straightforward, but, in the early stages may occasionally be confused with cardiac failure, the key differential features being the lack of pulsation in the jugular veins and the absence of tachycardia and gallop rhythm.

A chest X-ray usually shows tumour or lymph nodes in the right paratracheal area. The diagnosis can be confirmed by venography but this is not usually necessary unless thrombolysis, angioplasty and stenting are being considered (see below).

SVCO is sometimes regarded as an emergency requiring immediate treatment, but this is not necessary unless it is unusually severe with cerebral oedema, or if there is associated stridor. The symptoms and signs often stabilize after a few days and do not always go on getting worse, probably because adequate collaterals open up.

The majority of patients presenting with SVCO in the United Kingdom have lung cancer but there are other important causes such as malignant lymphoma and Hodgkin's disease. If the underlying diagnosis has not already been established, an attempt should be made to establish this first by bronchoscopy or, if necessary, mediastinoscopy (which can be carried out in this situation although there is a slightly increased risk of bleeding). This is particularly relevant in younger patients or non-smokers in whom a diagnosis other than lung cancer is more likely. It is also important to identify patients with SCLC.

Once the diagnosis has been made, the patient should be treated as appropriate with palliative radiotherapy or chemotherapy. It is usual for patients to get high dose corticosteroids (e.g. dexamethasone 16 mg a day), and although it is not clear whether this is really necessary, it may reduce inflammation, oedema or stridor, especially after radiotherapy starts.

The symptoms usually improve quite quickly after treatment starts but some patients do not get better. This can either be due to a lack of tumour response or be the result of permanent stricture or associated clot. For a few patients who are very troubled by the symptoms of SVCO and have either failed primary treatment or in whom the problem has recurred after radiotherapy it may be worth considering thrombolysis, angioplasty and stenting. These are invasive and complex procedures and should be reserved for patients who are otherwise fairly fit and seem to have a reasonable prognosis.

If this approach is thought to be appropriate, the diagnosis must be confirmed by venography. It is then usually necessary to carry out thrombolysis by infusion of streptokinase or urokinase for 24 to 48 hours through long intravenous catheters. Once the clot has been cleared a distinct area of stricture is often visible which can be stretched by balloon angioplasty, and it may then be possible to insert an expanding wire stent into the site of stricture to prevent it from recurring. Oral anticoagulants should then be continued for a few weeks.

STRIDOR

Stridor is one of the more distressing acute symptoms of lung cancer. It is caused by obstruction of the trachea, but can occur if one main stem bronchus is significantly obstructed in a patient with poor respiratory reserve.

The diagnosis can often be missed and should be specifically examined for. The patient is breathless and has noisy, stridulous breathing. The only differential diagnosis is between upper and lower airway obstruction and in a patient presenting for the first time it is essential to exclude a primary tumour in the larynx or pharynx. Provided the patient is fit enough the diagnosis should be confirmed by bronchoscopy and biopsy.

Treatment has to start promptly. Dexamethasone 12–16 mg daily may help reduce any associated oedema and should be given before radiotherapy, because corticosteroids seem to prevent the acute oedema that is sometimes induced by irradiation. If there is any suspicion of associated infection this should be treated. Palliative radiotherapy is usually the treatment of choice and it is probably prudent to give fractionated treatment (e.g. 20 Gy in five fractions) rather than large single fractions. The presence of stridor is not a contraindication to radical radiotherapy if the patient is otherwise fit enough and suitable (see Chapter 5) and can tolerate the inevitable delay in arranging a planned treatment. Patients with newly diagnosed SCLC should be treated with chemotherapy as the response is likely to be as quick as with radiotherapy.

Patients who are very distressed and significantly hypoxaemic should get supplementary oxygen, although care needs to be taken with high-concentration oxygen in patients with significant CO_2 retention. Patients with severe stridor may be helped by inhalation of an oxygen/helium mixture, which has a lower viscosity and flows more easily through the obstructed airway.

If the appropriate equipment and expertise are available it may be possible to enlarge the airway by laser therapy when there is endoluminal tumour rather than extrinsic compression. This may be a valuable technique to tide the patient over until more definitive treatment can start or when stridor recurs.

Recurrence of stridor after first-line treatment is common. It may still be possible to irradiate the patient, especially if the primary treatment was chemotherapy, but re-irradiation is often thought hazardous because of the risk of spinal cord damage. This hazard is probably more theoretical than real because the patient is unlikely to survive long enough (six to nine months) to run into the time of risk. It seems reasonable to explain the possible risk to the patient and then give additional fractionated treatment (20 Gy in five fractions). If the equipment is available, endoluminal brachytherapy may be very useful in this situation.

Very occasionally there are patients who are very fit with no evidence of metastases and with severe symptomatic stridor after maximum doses of radiotherapy. In this situation it may be possible to insert stents into the trachea and main stem bronchi.

If all else fails and the patient is very distressed by stridor, the only option is sedation with opiates and benzodiazepines.

DYSPNOEA

Dyspnoea is a common symptom of patients with bronchial carcinoma and can be caused by a combination of different factors:

- airway obstruction by tumour
- pleural effusion
- pericardial effusion
- infection
- underlying lung disease (usually chronic obstructive airways disease)
- other causes (e.g. pulmonary embolus, heart failure, anaemia)

It is therefore important to identify the cause of the dyspnoea before deciding the best management strategy.

When caused by tumour blocking a major airway, dyspnoea may improve after palliative radiotherapy or chemotherapy. However, it is one of the major symptoms of lung cancer that is the least well palliated. This is probably because of underlying chronic lung disease and also because if there is long-standing collapse and consolidation distal to the obstruction, the lung may not re-expand fully even if the airway is re-opened.

It is important to remember the value of oxygen therapy even though some patients with chronic lung disease may have CO_2 retention.

A fit patient with recurrent, symptomatic dyspnoea and definite endobronchial tumour in a proximal airway which has recurred after maximal doses of radiotherapy should be considered for laser treatment or endoluminal brachytherapy.

As with stridor there may come a time when all reasonable treatments have been tried and the dyspnoea is so disabling, that a small dose of opiate (e.g. morphine 10 mg, four- to six-hourly) may be helpful.

HAEMOPTYSIS

Haemoptysis is one of the cardinal symptoms of lung cancer and many patients experience it during the initial phase of their illness. It is a frightening symptom, but is usually intermittent and rarely a major source of blood loss. It responds well to palliative radiotherapy.

The main problems with haemoptysis are encountered in patients with recurrent disease. It may be possible to repeat palliative radiotherapy, and haemoptysis is a good indication for endobronchial brachytherapy if facilities are available. Laser treatment may also be an option in this situation.

It is important to ensure the patient is not on aspirin or other non-steroidal anti-inflammatory drugs. When all other treatments have failed, it is usual to give ethamsylate (500 mg q.d.s.) although its effectiveness in this situation is uncertain.

Massive haemoptysis can be a rapidly fatal, terminal event and is usually due to erosion into a major blood vessel by tumour or radiation necrosis. It is important to give adequate sedation as quickly as possible because little else can be done.

COUGH

Cough can be a very troublesome symptom. It is usually due to tumour in the airways but may be caused by intercurrent infection or radiation pneumonitis. A severe cough associated with eating and drinking suggests a broncho-oesophageal fistula.

Simple anti-tussives (e.g. codeine linctus) may be helpful, but some patients may need a stronger opiate such as methadone linctus or oral morphine. Palliative radiotherapy is often effective in improving severe cough.

BRONCHO-OESOPHAGEAL FISTULA

Broncho-oesophageal fistula occasionally occurs when a tumour mass invades both oesophagus and a main bronchus and there is either spontaneous or treatment-related (usually radiotherapy) necrosis. The clinical picture is characteristic, with recurrent chest infections and fits of coughing whenever the patient drinks. There is usually associated dysphagia and rapid weight loss because eating and drinking are difficult if not impossible.

Management is difficult and usually unsatisfactory. The fistula is unlikely to close and surgery is generally not appropriate. If the fistula is small, it may be possible to pass a fine-bore nasogastric tube either blind or under endoscopic control and to feed the patient that way but liquid may still get into the airway and cause problems. A few patients may be suitable for an oesophageal stent but this may be difficult to place and retain in position. A feeding gastrotomy tube can be considered but is not often appropriate for patients with terminal disease. Sedation may be the only appropriate management and a continuous infusion pump with hyoscine may help control secretions.

PAIN CONTROL

Pain is such a common problem that it is worth briefly outlining the principles of good pain management.

The first important step is to make as precise a diagnosis of the cause or causes of the patient's pain as possible. The commoner causes are as follows:

- Primary tumour invasion of parietal pleura, mediastinum, chest wall, rib or vertebral body.
- Primary tumour invasion of intercostal nerve or brachial plexus.
- Bone metastases, particularly if there is pathological fracture.
- Liver metastasis if there is capsular distension or invasion, or haemorrhage.
- Other sites of metastasis (e.g. skin and adrenal glands).
- Post-thoracotomy pain
- Facial pain

Clearly, the first treatment of choice for all these problems (except post-thoracotomy pain) is directed specifically at the tumour (surgery, radiotherapy or chemotherapy) and pain can respond dramatically. The pain of bone metastases has an inflammatory component and may be helped by a non-steroidal anti-inflammatory drug. Unfortunately the common problem is that of increasing pain due to recurrent tumour and so it is often necessary to resort to increasingly strong analgesics.

The important principles of analgesic prescription for patients with tumour-related pain are:

- Become familiar with one range of analgesics (non-opiate, mild opiate, strong opiate).
- Make sure the patient takes the drugs regularly to keep themselves pain-free.
- Escalate the strength and dose of analgesic rapidly to get on top of the pain.

- Do not be afraid of using adequate doses of strong opiates even in patients with chronic lung disease.
- Always give regular laxatives with any opiate.

The advent of morphine in tablet form for both immediate (Sevredol) and sustained release (MST Continus) and in a range of strengths, has made the prescribing of strong opiates much easier and has reduced the need for liquid solutions which are inconvenient, difficult to give accurately and have a short shelf-life. When starting a patient on morphine it is usually best to give immediate-release tablets regularly every four hours with instructions to the patient, carer or nurses to increase the dose if the pain is not adequately controlled during each four-hour period. Once good analgesia has been established, the total dose over 24 hours can be added up, divided by two and that dose given by sustained release, twice daily. The pharmacology of these tablets is such that, unless there is particular reason to think that metabolism is abnormal, it is unnecessary to give them more often, and if pain control is not sustained for the full 12 hours, it is better to increase the dose than to go to 8-hour dose intervals. There are occasional patients who seem to metabolize the tablets more quickly and in whom better pain control is achieved by 8-hourly doses.

Some patients may find it difficult to manage tablets especially in high doses and, if the prognosis is very poor, it may be necessary to give opiates through a continuous subcutaneous infusion from a syringe driver pump.

Opiates do, of course have their problems:

- Constipation is universal and often very distressing. Giving regular softeners (e.g. lactulose) and stimulants (e.g. Co-danthramer) is essential but some patients will need intermittent enemata.
- Nausea and vomiting often occur especially when opiates are first given. In most patients they respond to simple anti-emetics and tend to improve after the first week or so. But some patients may find this to be a major problem and not be able to tolerate morphine. Changing to another opiate may sometimes help, as may giving it parenterally in a syringe-driver combined with a suitable anti-emetic (e.g. methotrimeprazine or haloperidol).
- Drowsiness is common especially when the dose is increased and susceptible patients may also become confused. As with nausea, it may improve after a week to ten days, but some patients may prefer to have a bit more pain and stay alert.
- Hallucinations and nightmares are occasionally distressing and are more common with the weaker, partial agonist analogues (e.g. pethidine and pentazocine), which really have no place in the management of chronic cancer pain.
- Troublesome myoclonus can occur when very high doses of opiate (above 500 mg of morphine a day) are given. It may be helped by benzodiazepines, which will, of course, increase sedation.

Many patients are apprehensive about starting on strong opiates. They may see it as a sign of a poor prognosis and imminent death, may have fears of becoming addicted, over-sedated or losing control or may perceive dependence on opiates as a sign of weakness. Simple reassurance is usually enough and patients can be told quite honestly that if they are taking opiates for pain they are very unlikely to become addicted and that if the pain responds to other measures (such as radiotherapy) the dose can easily be reduced.

Some patients have pain that is apparently opiate-resistant. The commonest cause of this is neurogenic pain from nerve infiltration (e.g. intercostal nerve or brachial plexus). It may be helped by tricyclic anti-depressants or mexiletine (150 mg daily up to 300 mg eight-hourly), or physical treatment such as acupuncture and trans-cutaneous nerve stimulation. Anti-convulsants (e.g. carbamazepine 100 mg t.d.s.) may help if the pain has a lancinating character. Nerve-blocking procedures — either temporary or permanent — may eventually be needed. These are best done in a specialist pain clinic but it is worth remembering that patients can get considerable (and surprisingly long-lasting) relief of localized chest-wall pain by a simple intercostal nerve block with bupivacaine.

Psychological distress may also make pain more severe and not respond to opiates. It is worth exploring problems with the patient and, if appropriate, prescribing an anti-depressant or major tranquilliser (see Chapter 12).

ANOREXIA

Anorexia and weight loss occur frequently in all types of lung cancer and may be severe even in the absence of metastases. The cause is not entirely clear but they may be associated with the production of interleukin-6. The symptoms usually get worse as the disease progresses, particularly if there are liver metastases. They usually improve with successful primary treatment of the tumour (even with chemotherapy), but can be a distressing, obvious reminder of the cancer in the later stages.

Simple dietary advice may be very helpful in ensuring that the patient maintains a reasonable calorie intake. Quite a range of palatable dietary supplements is available, some of which can be prescribed.

Corticosteroids (e.g. prednisolone 30 mg daily) are often given and can be very helpful for some patients. If there is no benefit after two or three weeks there is probably no point in continuing.

Recently there has been interest in giving progestagens (e.g. megesterol acetate 160 mg b.d.). They may be effective, but there is no evidence from controlled studies that they offer any advantages in efficacy or side-effects over corticosteroids.

PLEURAL EFFUSION

Pleural effusion can occur if there is pleural involvement by tumour and is particularly frequent in patients with mesothelioma (see Chapter 14).

It can produce distressing breathlessness especially when large enough to cause mediastinal shift. The diagnosis is usually obvious clinically and on chest X-ray but occasionally (especially if there has been previous aspiration and attempted pleurodesis) ultrasound may help to localize a loculated effusion or confirm that there is not just pleural thickening.

Tube drainage is probably better than needle aspiration because the rate can be controlled and it is easier to achieve complete drainage with less risk of producing a pneumothorax, but does entail a hospital stay of at least 24 hours. There are simple modern catheter systems that are easier to insert than the traditional tubes.

If there is underlying lung collapse it may be difficult to achieve complete drainage and re-expansion of the lung and so the patient is unlikely to benefit symptomatically from prolonged drainage.

Pleurodesis should be carried out once all fluid has been drained, in order to prevent recurrence. Tetracycline is probably safer and as effective as using cytotoxic agents like bleomycin or mustine (which probably work by producing inflammation rather than through any anti-tumour effect). The technique is as follows:

- Establish by chest X-ray that drainage is complete
- Give prophylactic analgesics (e.g. morphine 10 mg or diclofenac 50 mg)
- Instil 20 ml of 1% lignocaine and 5 ml normal saline down intercostal tube
- Clamp the tube for 20 minutes
- Instil tetracycline 1 G in 50 ml of saline and 10 ml normal saline
- Leave for 2 hours
- Allow fluid to drain out and remove the tube.

PERICARDIAL EFFUSION

Involvement of the pericardium by tumour can lead to the development of a pericardial effusion and, eventually, cardiac tamponade. Pericardial effusion should be suspected if there is progressive enlargement of the heart shadow on chest X-ray, particularly if it has a 'globular' shape, in the absence of signs of heart failure. The diagnosis can be confirmed by cardiac ultrasound.

Pericardial aspiration under ultrasound control is the first-line management, especially in patients with tamponade. This can be repeated as necessary. Instillation of sclerosing agents such as tetracycline can be tried but is of unproven benefit.

Patients with persisting problems who are otherwise fit may need a permanent pericardial 'window' created to drain the effusion into the pleural space.

ASCITES

Troublesome ascites sometimes occurs in patients with lung cancer either due to peritoneal metastases or secondary to liver failure and hypo-albuminaemia. If it is causing uncomfortable abdominal distension it is worth draining it. There is no place for instilling cytotoxic agents or tetracycline into the peritoneal cavity.

SPINAL CORD COMPRESSION

Spinal cord compression usually results from extradural compression in the thoracic spine, either by direct tumour extension from the primary, from mediastinal lymph nodes or from vertebral body metastases, or as a result of pathological collapse of a vertebra. Rarely it may be caused by intramedullary spinal metastasis, particularly in SCLC. The differential diagnosis includes radiation myelopathy (see Chapter 5), non-metastatic degeneration (see Chapter 10) and all the other non-malignant causes of myelopathy.

The early symptoms and signs are easily overlooked but it is a condition that should be suspected in any patient who complains of leg weakness, difficulty in walking or of a sudden onset of urinary symptoms. The only chance of improvement is if the diagnosis is made early and, once sphincter control has been lost, significant recovery is very unlikely.

Careful examination usually reveals muscle weakness, changes in the reflexes and a sensory level. It is important to remember that cauda equina compression can give a flaccid paresis and sensory changes in the sacral dermatomes which must always be tested. When there is any doubt about urinary function it is best to catheterize the patient early to look for residual urine and symptomless retention.

If the underlying cause is obvious (such as vertebral body collapse at an appropriate level) then dexamethasone 16 mg a day should be started and the patient sent for urgent radiotherapy. If there is any doubt about the cause, the neurosurgeons should be consulted and a myelogram (or MR scan) carried out to establish the diagnosis and define the site of the lesion.

Radiotherapy should be started as soon as possible. A dose of 20 Gy in five fractions is adequate with a field that generously covers the known or suspected site of compression. It is important to remember that the actual lesion is usually higher than the neurological signs would suggest and there is the possibility of multiple lesions, particularly with intramedullary deposits.

If there is any prospect of recovery, physiotherapy should be started early to maintain residual function and to prevent contractures.

MENINGEAL DISEASE

Meningeal tumour deposits occasionally occur, usually from SCLC. The neurological symptoms and signs are often vague and confusing and typically consist of widespread nerve root motor weakness or sensory abnormalities and pain. The diagnosis should be established by myelography, MR scan and cerebrospinal fluid (CSF) analysis. The CSF may contain obvious tumour cells but, if not, the presence of low glucose and high protein levels is characteristic.

Meningeal disease is difficult to treat. If the patient has SCLC and has not previously received methotrexate as part of the systemic chemotherapy, it may be possible to give this drug intrathecally (up to 12 mg, twice weekly, until the CSF is clear). If localised deposits are causing local symptoms it may also be possible to give palliative radiotherapy.

HYPERTROPHIC PULMONARY OSTEOARTHROPATHY (HPOA)

Some patients with finger clubbing develop an associated arthropathy, mainly affecting wrist, ankle and knee joints. This has a characteristic radiological appearance with calcifying periostitis near the joint.

The cause of this condition, as with finger clubbing itself, is obscure. It is less common in patients with SCLC but otherwise is not particularly associated with any histological type of lung cancer, size or site of tumour. It usually resolves if the tumour is completely resected and often gets a little better after palliative radiotherapy to the primary. Otherwise it has to be managed symptomatically with non-steroidal anti-inflammatory drugs and stronger analgesics. Injection of corticosteroids into troublesome joints may also be helpful.

FACIAL PAIN

Some patients with lung cancer experience facial pain, usually on the same side as the tumour. This can be the presenting symptom of the disease and some patients with chronic facial pain, particularly of the so-called 'atypical' kind turn out to have a lung tumour.

The pain is typically constant with a 'deep' or 'boring' character radiating up into the neck, jaw, pinna and side of face. Involvement of the pinna is said to be characteristic and it has been suggested that it may be due to involvement of the vagus in the mediastinum referred via the auricular branch.

Palliative radiotherapy to the primary often improves the pain, sometimes dramatically. It may be resistant to opiates but be helped by anti-convulsants.

HORNER'S SYNDROME

Horner's syndrome with unilateral enophthalmos, miosis, partial ptosis and loss of sweating on one side of the face can result from tumour involvement of the sympathetic chain in the upper mediastinum and commonly occurs with Pancoast tumours (see Chapter 5). It rarely causes severe symptoms but the increased sweating on the other side of the face can be worrying and inconvenient. It does not usually improve with palliative radiotherapy but patients are often helped by a simple explanation and reassurance.

KEY POINTS

- Superior vena cava obstruction is a common complication of lung cancer which may be overlooked in the early stages. First-line management is with corticosteroids and radiotherapy, or chemotherapy, but thrombolysis and stenting should be considered for some patients.
- Stridor is an unpleasant symptom requiring urgent treatment with corticosteriods and palliative radiotherapy.
- It is important to establish a clear diagnosis in a patient with increasing dyspnoea.
- Intractable cough and recurrent chest infection may be due to broncho-oesophageal fistula.
- Adequate pain control may require escalating, regular doses of opiates.
- Anti-emetics and laxatives should always be prescribed with opiates.
- Corticosteroids may help anorexia.
- Complete drainage of a pleural effusion is essential before pleurodesis is attempted.

FURTHER READING

Doyle D., Hanks G.W.C., Macdonald N. (Eds) (1993) *Oxford Textbook of Palliative Medicine.* Oxford: Oxford Medical Publications.

11 PARANEOPLASTIC
NEUROLOGICAL PROBLEMS

Patients with lung cancer quite often present with neurological symptoms and signs. They are particularly at risk of developing cerebral metastases, spinal cord compression or cerebrovascular events due to smoking-related vascular disease. Non-bacterial thrombotic (marantic) endocarditis may occasionally occur and cause emboli which lead to complex neurological signs or a progressive encephalopathy.

In addition, a variety of paraneoplastic syndromes have been described in association with lung cancer and it has been estimated that 1–2% of patients will have one form or another. It is important, however, to exclude potentially treatable causes for the clinical findings before attributing them to a paraneoplastic syndrome.

CEREBELLAR SYNDROME

A cerebellar syndrome, characterized by symmetrical bilateral cerebellar dysfunction with ataxia, dysarthria and hypotonia may occur and anti-neuronal antibodies have been demonstrated in some patients. There are reports of improvement following successful treatment of the underlying tumour and after plasmapheresis.

CEREBRAL SYNDROMES

The commonest cerebral abnormality associated with lung cancer is a progressive dementia usually associated with a generalized slowing of the electro-encephalogram. Research has suggested the cause to be a proliferation of endothelial cells in blood vessels caused by secretion of an angiogenic peptide by tumour cells. Occasional responses to high-dose steroids have been reported.

Visual disturbances may occur with optic neuritis and there may be unilateral or bilateral scotomas and papilloedema. This is most commonly associated with SCLC.

A syndrome of progressive dementia and ataxia has been seen in some long-term survivors after treatment for SCLC and has been attributed to the late effects of cranial irradiation (see Chapter 7).

SPINAL CORD AND PERIPHERAL NERVE ABNORMALITIES

A syndrome similar to motor neurone disease has been described, comprising widespread lower motor-neurone muscle weakness, spasticity, muscle atrophy and hyperreflexia.

Lung cancer may also be associated with a devastating syndrome of a rapidly ascending motor and sensory paralysis (subacute necrotic myelopathy) which may result in respiratory failure and death within weeks. There are anecdotal reports of responses to intrathecal steroids in this situation.

Peripheral neuropathy can occur and this may be either acute or chronic. Combined sensory and motor deficits may steadily progress and lead to paralysis but the symptoms and signs frequently have a more fluctuating course. There is often only minimal improvement with treatment of the underlying tumour.

Degeneration of dorsal root ganglia leading to a pure sensory neuropathy can be associated with several types of tumours but most frequently with lung cancer. Distal sensory loss occurs with preservation of muscle tone and strength. In some patients the syndrome may precede the detection of the primary neoplasm. It appears likely that there is an autoimmune cause for this syndrome, with the production of antibodies directed against peripheral nerve myelin. Unfortunately, treatment of the underlying tumour rarely produces a clinical improvement.

AUTONOMIC NEUROPATHY

An autonomic neuropathy causing postural hypotension and bladder and bowel abnormalities has been described in association with lung cancer.

EATON–LAMBERT SYNDROME

The Eaton–Lambert syndrome is particularly associated with small cell carcinoma of the bronchus. Muscle weakness and fatigue, dysarthria, dysphagia and visual disturbances are features and, unlike myasthenia gravis, exercise is associated with increasing muscle strength and there is a negative response to Tensilon. Electromyography may be useful in confirming the diagnosis.

Combination chemotherapy to treat the underlying tumour may be associated with improvement in the syndrome. Symptomatic benefit in patients who do not improve with chemotherapy may be obtained with the use of guanidine hydrochloride 250 mg three or four times a day.

POLYMYOSITIS

Polymyositis presents as a progressive painful weakness mainly in proximal muscle groups, with diminished reflexes and no sensory abnormalities. Muscle enzymes are elevated and there are characteristic changes on muscle biopsy. It can be associated with a dermatitis (dermatomyositis), the magenta rash characteristically occurring on the face, particularly around the eyes, the hands and feet.

The myositis may precede the clinical presentation of the cancer. Improvement may occur after treating the underlying tumour and corticosteroids may sometimes help.

KEY POINT

- Paraneoplastic neurological syndromes are uncommon and other causes for the symptoms (e.g. metastases and drug toxicity) should be carefully sought.

FURTHER READING

Bunn Jr. P., Ridgway E.C. (1993) Paraneoplastic Syndromes. In *Cancer: Principles and Practice of Oncology.* 4th edn. Edited by De Vita, Hellman and Rosenberg. Philadelphia: J.B. Lippincott and Co.

12 COMMUNICATION AND PSYCHOLOGICAL PROBLEMS

As with all serious illnesses, the problems of patients with lung cancer are not entirely physical. Almost all patients will experience considerable psychological and emotional stress during the course of their illness. They will probably be frightened by the initial symptoms and investigations and be upset by the confirmation of the diagnosis and its life-threatening implications. They may have to go through major surgery or toxic chemotherapy both of which can cause psychological as well as physical problems, or come to terms with the knowledge of incurability. Finally, many will have to face the reality of rapid physical decline and approaching death.

Coping with all these problems will be hard for all but the most robust and phlegmatic patients, but most people do manage to achieve a degree of psychological adaptation. These stresses will also affect the patient's family and they too will need help and support.

It is essential that all professionals who are involved in the physical care of patients with lung cancer have some skills in lessening these traumas, in recognising the problems and in helping to deal with them. It seems probable that good and honest communication throughout the illness will help patients to adapt. These skills, however, are not well taught and not often acknowledged, let alone valued in the technological milieu of modern medicine. The increase in the provision of hospice care and of trained nurse counsellors has improved the overall amount of such care available but does not lessen our own responsibilities to be sensitive to and to respond to the patients' psychological needs.

In this chapter we will discuss some of the most common areas of difficulty and give some simple advice on management. However this is not an area that lends itself well to didactic written instruction and we would urge anyone who recognises their own shortcomings to look for some professional teaching, which is increasingly available. Contrary to widespread belief these skills can be taught and learnt and are not somehow innate.

COMMUNICATION

Good communication is essential for managing patients with lung cancer at all stages of their illness and the better the communication the more likely they are to give important information about themselves, adapt psychologically and cooperate with treatment. As a result they may be less anxious or depressed and less likely to complain about their care.

There are a number of important basic points that can help.

- **Get the setting right**. Finding a quiet, private place with comfortable chairs and good acoustics is very helpful. Wards and outpatient clinics rarely attain this ideal.

116

- **Avoid interruptions**. Unplug the telephone, switch off the bleeper and do not allow people to walk in. This is also difficult to achieve in most hospitals.
- **Get your body language right**. Most patients find doctors in white coats frightening to some extent and this can be made worse by the way the doctor behaves. Be friendly and open, maintain eye-contact and do not hide behind desks, piles of case-notes or folded arms. Try to sit at the same level or slightly lower than the patient.
- **Get your language and pacing right**. Use words and descriptions that the patient is likely to understand, avoiding jargon and technical terms, and speak more slowly and clearly than feels natural.
- **Check understanding**. Check fairly frequently that you are being understood by asking if everything is clear and whether more details are wanted. This gives the patient a chance to direct the way the conversation goes, to ask for more information or reject the offer.
- **Notice** the patient's emotional reactions and body language and respond to them as appropriate (see below).
- Make sure that the most important things are said at the beginning of the interview as they are then more likely to be remembered. Repeat things if you feel they need particular emphasis and perhaps reiterate them at the end of the conversation.
- **Be consistent** in what you say on different occasions and, as far as possible when talking to the patient and his relatives (see below). Record the important points of what you have said so that others know what has been said and can also be consistent.

BREAKING BAD NEWS

Anyone looking after patients with lung cancer has to give a lot of bad news to patients and relatives and needs to become good at doing it gently, honestly and sympathetically. There are a few hints that may make this difficult job easier.

- Find out first what the patient already knows or suspects. This may sometimes shorten the whole conversation when the patient says something like: 'It's cancer, isn't it?'. Many know or suspect the truth even if it has never been explicitly stated and find confirmation a relief.
- Ask the patient if he or she wants to know more about their illness and treatment. Most patients do want to be fully informed.
- Pace what you say. It is a good idea to give the patient some warning that what you are about to say is bad news. Then give the actual information bit by bit, pausing frequently to allow the information to be absorbed.
- Encourage and allow time for questions as you go along, and check that what you are saying is really being understood. There is a natural tendency to rush things especially when the conversation is tricky.
- Be prepared and allow for emotional reactions (see below).
- Be honest at all times. If a patient asks a direct question, give as truthful an answer as you can. Do not resort to inappropriate reassurances; although it may make

everything more comfortable for you and the patient at the time, it is likely to cause problems in the future when things go wrong.
- Try to give something positive along with the bad news, a clear plan for treatment or assurances that unpleasant symptoms such as pain can be controlled, for instance.
- Allow for the fact that much of what is said may not be remembered and that it may be necessary to go back later and repeat it. It is sometimes very obvious when someone 'switches off' and it is probably not worth giving more information at that time, though it may be helpful to explore their anxiety and emotions.
- It may be helpful to have one close relative with the patient at the time that bad news is given. Although it sometimes makes the conversation more difficult to direct and some patients may feel inhibited in what they are prepared to say, there are advantages in having someone else to remember what is said and to provide support.

We should no longer be afraid of using the word 'cancer' with patients. It is a term that everyone understands whereas words like 'growth', 'tumour' and 'malignant', which can be used to soften the impact, may in fact confuse some patients or give them an inappropriate false reassurance. Most patients do want to know exactly what is wrong with them (and suspect the true diagnosis anyway) and it is wrong to deny them that knowledge on the probably false assumption that they will not 'cope'. Patients who genuinely do not want to know usually make it clear early in any conversation and even if they have not done so and are given 'unwelcome' information, they may block it out and 'forget'. Denial is an important and powerful mental defence mechanism.

COPING WITH EMOTIONAL REACTIONS

Emotional reactions are frequent and entirely natural and we all need to be able to cope with them. The common reaction is distress and tears, but sometimes patients become angry either with something or someone specific or else in an unfocused, general way. The emotional issues may be too complex and difficult to be dealt with simply, in which case skilled professional counselling may be needed, but it is important to try to partly resolve or at least clarify them at the time.
A few pointers may be helpful in dealing with emotionally distressed patients.

- Acknowledge and respond to the patients' emotional reactions, whether openly expressed or implicit in body language, and do not ignore them or brush them aside. They often feel ashamed of their reactions and embarrassed, but acknowledgement, by some simple phrase like 'I can see this must be upsetting for you', gives them permission to open up further if they want to.
- Give the patients time and silence, so that they can either collect themselves or else talk more if they want. Do not try to rush on and give more information until the reaction has been at least superficially resolved.
- Try to find out if there are particular things that are upsetting them. This may

reveal important information about social problems, previous experience of cancer in the family or misconceptions about the illness or treatment. These may be issues that can be dealt with very simply by explanation or reassurance, or may lead on to a referral for social support etc.

- Do not be afraid of physical contact. Shaking hands on first meeting the patient or relative is more than a social nicety and helps to break down barriers. Touching the patient on the hand or shoulder during emotional parts of the interview, provided it is a spontaneous-seeming gesture, can be an effective non-verbal way of expressing empathy and support.
- Try to end the interview on a positive note and offer them another opportunity to talk later. They may also want time alone or with a nurse before leaving.

DISCUSSING THE PROGNOSIS

Discussing the prognosis with lung cancer patients is often very difficult purely because the outlook for most is so bad. Not many patients will ask about it at the first interview, but many will eventually want to do so, especially if some trust and rapport have been built up.

It is wrong to attempt to give any precise time because it is always likely to be inaccurate, and yet the patient or the relatives may fix on it as a certainty. The fictional image of the doctor giving a patient 'six months to live' is so deeply engrained in our collective folklore that patients and relatives find it hard to accept that we cannot give an accurate prognosis.

It is, however, important to emphasize the seriousness of the illness and the uncertainty of the outcome. It may be appropriate to say that the condition is unlikely to be cured, although it may be controlled for some time. If pushed to give a time limit (and some patients may have very genuine reasons for wanting to know what to expect) it is probably best to be non-specific but as truthful as possible with phrases like 'months rather than years' or 'weeks rather than months'.

TALKING TO RELATIVES

It is an essential part of the care of patients to talk to their relatives. All the general points made above apply but there are some specific issues.

In the past it was commonplace for the relatives of patients with cancer to be told the diagnosis before the patient (who often was not told at all) and this led to a number of problems. First of all there was the awkward scene of relatives being ushered covertly into the ward office at visiting time without being seen by the patient. Secondly, the relatives often asked, with the best motive of protecting the patient, for him not to be told the truth, which could lead to problems. The situation when a relative has been told explicitly while the patient has not but suspects and neither will talk frankly to the other, may be very difficult and distressing to sustain. This kind of practice should no longer occur, unless there are exceptional circumstances.

It is an ethical principle that medical information should not be disclosed to a third party (even a close relative) without the patient's specific permission, and this principle applies equally to patients with lung cancer. It is usually best if the patient and a relative are talked to together on at least one occasion, but there are often situations when it is easier if the relatives are spoken to alone. Some patients do not want to know everything and sometimes the relatives should be given more explicit details of the illness and the prognosis than the patient. It should, however, be the exception (and there may be rare occasions when it is appropriate) that this is done without the patient's permission.

WRITTEN INFORMATION AND TAPES

Because it is difficult to give and receive complex information, especially in an interview that has a strong emotional content, it may be helpful to give patients written information about the disease or treatment. There are a number of pamphlets and booklets, produced by hospitals and charitable organizations, which can be bought for use. It is important to ensure that the information is accurate and applicable, and if parts are not relevant to a particular patient, to point that out.

Another technique that is helpful to patients is for important parts of the interview to be recorded and the patient to be given the tape. It can then be played over at home, other relatives can hear what has been said and the patient can pick up any information that was missed the first time. The tape, once returned, can be used to assess one's own performance or be used for teaching.

ANXIETY

Anxiety is an inevitable accompaniment of serious illness and its treatment. For most patients simple reassurance and explanation is enough to help them cope and draw on their own resources and, over a period of time, psychological adaptation to the knowledge that they have cancer takes place.

Some patients, however, usually with a pre-morbid personality and a history of phobic reactions, may develop phobic problems about aspects of their treatment, such as coming to hospital for radiotherapy or chemotherapy. These patients need to be recognised early on and referred for professional psychological help because they can be helped by specific desensitization and relaxation techniques.

It is also important to recognise the patients who do not adapt psychologically and remain severely anxious. They are usually obvious by their behaviour and conversation, but some may just complain of the symptoms of arousal, such as sweating, tremor, restlessness and inability to sleep. They may be helped in the short term by benzodiazepines but will also need professional counselling or psychiatric referral.

DEPRESSION

It is not surprising that many patients with lung cancer become depressed. In most cases this is not severe and may improve with simple reassurance or following an obvious improvement in symptoms and general well-being as a result of treatment.

Some patients do develop a more severe and long-lasting depression. Many probably go undetected in the normal clinic because they will tend to hide their true feelings, put on a front and not want to 'bother the doctor'. Even when looking out for it, it can be quite difficult to establish the diagnosis as many of the cardinal symptoms such as sleep disturbance, retardation, loss of concentration and anorexia can occur as a result of the illness or its treatment (especially if opiates are given). The key symptoms in this situation may be loss of motivation and of the sense of enjoyment.

Although these patients may be helped by the chance to talk about their feelings, problems and fears, or by professional counselling and support, those with moderate or severe symptoms should be treated with anti-depressants.

ACUTE CONFUSIONAL STATE

Patients with lung cancer may become acutely confused for a number of reasons, the most frequent of which are:

- Chest infection and hypoxia
- Hypercalcaemia
- Hyponatremia
- Opiates
- Brain metastases
- High dose corticosteroids

It is important to make a precise diagnosis and treat the patient appropriately.

KEY POINTS

- Good communication is an essential part of good clinical care.
- Give patients and relatives the information that they want and need rather than what you think they want. Be as honest and straightforward as possible and do not be afraid to use the word 'cancer' or to talk about the prognosis.
- Try to give positive information and advice along with any bad news.
- Try to deal with emotional reactions at the time.
- Anxiety and depression are common reactions to illness and may require specific treatment.

FURTHER READING

Buckman R. (1992) *How to Break Bad News*. London: Papermac.
Hughes J. (1987) *Cancer and Emotion*. Chichester: John Wiley and Sons.
Fallowfield L. (1993) *Giving Sad and Bad News*. Lancet, **341**, 476–478.

13 CARCINOID TUMOURS

Approximately 12% of all carcinoid tumours arise in the lung and they account for 1–2% of all primary lung cancers. They are thought to arise from cells of the diffuse neuroendocrine system (Feyrter cells) which are present in the bronchial epthelium. Unlike foregut carcinoids, bronchial carcinoids rarely give the argentaffin reaction.

PATHOLOGY (see Chapter 4)

CLINICAL PRESENTATION

Bronchial carcinoid tumours are most often found as an incidental abnormality on a routine chest X-ray, but up to 20% of patients may present with a cough, an unresolving chest infection or with symptoms suggestive of the carcinoid syndrome.

LOCALIZATION OF THE PRIMARY TUMOUR

In the majority of patients with bronchial carcinoids, the primary tumour can be seen on a chest X-ray, or on a CT or MR scan of the thorax. Endobronchial tumours are sometimes seen at bronchoscopy. They are usually slow growing and may ultimately produce major airway obstruction and distal atelectasis, but hilar lymphadenopathy is rare. Liver metastases may be demonstrated by CT scanning, ultrasonography or angiography.

Over 50% of primary and metastatic carcinoid tumours may be localized by scanning with ^{131}I radiolabelled MIBG (meta-iodo benzyl guanidine). The synthetic somatostatin analogue, iodinated octreotide, has recently also been shown to localize a high percentage of carcinoid tumours and is increasingly used to image both the primary tumour and its metastases.

MANAGEMENT

Approximately 80% of patients with a primary bronchial carcinoid tumour will not have overt metastases at the time of diagnosis, and should be offered surgery. This should be curative and result in a five-year survival rate of more than 90%. Even if regional nodes are involved, provided they can be removed, long term survival is possible and five-year survival rates of around 70% can be achieved.

The potential for cure is less when there are distant metastases, but even so about 10% of patients may survive for five years.

Once metastases have occurred, there are several options for management. Isolated liver metastases may be resectable and several series have suggested useful benefit from this procedure, with median survival times of five years from excision and, for patients with the carcinoid syndrome, symptomatic benefit. Alternatively, embolization through the hepatic artery may be effective if the liver metastases are few and the blood supply discrete. Radiotherapy to sites of symptomatic bone and skin metastases may be of value and may also be used for inoperable intrathoracic primary tumours which are causing symptoms. Radiation doses of 45–50 Gy over four or five weeks are generally recommended.

The role of chemotherapy in the treatment of malignant bronchial carcinoid tumours is uncertain. Several agents produce response rates of up to 30% in metastatic disease and these include 5-fluorouracil, doxorubicin, cisplatin, etoposide and cyclophosphamide. Streptozotocin was often used in the past but has significant toxicity and should be avoided. There is evidence that bronchial carcinoid tumours may respond to treatment better than tumours arising in the gastrointestinal tract, but the routine use of chemotherapy should be avoided unless patients fail to respond to less toxic procedures and are becoming increasingly symptomatic from metastatic disease.

CARCINOID SYNDROME

Carcinoid tumours can produce a variety of biologically active compounds including ACTH, somatostatin, insulin, growth hormone, calcitonin, vasoactive intestinal peptide (VIP) and other peptides, as well as 5-hydroxytryptamine, histamine and bradykinin (see below). These may all contribute to the features of the carcinoid syndrome: a constellation of symptoms including flushing attacks, diarrhoea, wheeze, pellagroid skin lesions and cardiac abnormalities. This most commonly occurs when carcinoids arising in the gut metastasize to the liver. It is quite rare in bronchial carcinoids and is usually also the result of liver metastases.

Facial flushing is the most common feature and is characterised by the sudden onset of erythema in the face, neck and upper half of the body sometimes accompanied by palpitations, pruritus and facial oedema. These episodes tend to last longer with bronchial carcinoids than with tumours arising in the gut and may sometimes go on for a few hours. After several episodes of flushing, the skin may become permanently erythematous.

There may also be excessive salivation and associated episodes of diarrhoea and hypertension. The diarrhoea may be profound with up to 30 episodes per day and may be associated with severe abdominal discomfort and steatorrhoea.

Endocardial fibrosis, predominantly affecting the right side of the heart, may result in heart failure. Typically, the tricuspid valve is involved, leading to tricuspid regurgitation but the pulmonary valve may also be affected. It is very unusual for changes to occur in the valves on the left side of the heart.

Other less common features of the carcinoid syndrome include arthralgia, confusion and retroperitoneal fibrosis which may lead to ureteric obstruction. Impotence is a common complaint in men.

BIOCHEMICAL PATHWAYS

The carcinoid syndrome occurs when the tumour drains hormones directly into the systemic circulation. Carcinoids arising in the gut require the presence of liver metastases to be associated with the carcinoid syndrome because hormones from the primary tumour drain into the portal venous system, but bronchial carcinoids may occasionally produce the syndrome without metastases.

A variety of bioactive molecules have been implicated in causing the symptoms. Tryptophan is first converted to 5-hydroxytryptophan and this is then converted to 5-hydroxytryptamine, also called serotonin, which is thought to be responsible for some of the major symptoms including diarrhoea. Serotonin may be stored in neurosecretory tumour granules or released into the circulation where it is mostly converted into 5-hydroxyindole acetic acid (5-HIAA), which can be detected in the urine. Occasionally there is a deficiency of the enzyme which converts 5-hydroxytryptophan to serotonin and the former is produced in excessive amounts and secreted into the blood, but the plasma levels of serotonin and the urinary levels of 5-HIAA are normal.

Although flushing was originally thought to be due to serotonin, it has been found that serotonin antagonists such as methysergide do not prevent it, and so other vasoactive agents including bradykinin, histamine and prostaglandins have been implicated. It seems likely, however, that serotonin is responsible for the diarrhoea associated with carcinoid syndrome and its effect seems to be induced by increasing gut motility and reducing fat absorption. Serotonin may also produce bronchospasm and be involved in the fibrosis of the heart valves.

DIAGNOSIS OF THE CARCINOID SYNDROME

When the carcinoid syndrome is suspected, the diagnosis can be confirmed by demonstrating increased levels of serotonin or its metabolites in the urine. Measurement of 5-HIAA levels in a 24-hour urine collection is the best initial investigation, with levels above 8 mg/24 hours suggesting the diagnosis. Falsely elevated urinary 5-HIAA levels may be found in patients with malabsorption states, in those eating serotonin-rich foods (bananas, nuts) or taking a variety of medications including aspirin and l-dopa, and so serotonin levels may also need to be measured in urine and platelets.

Approximately 75% of patients with the carcinoid syndrome will be diagnosed from measurements of urinary serotonin or its metabolites, and for the remaining patients a variety of investigations have been suggested including measurement of plasma levels of substance P, serum chromogranin levels and observation of the development of symptoms after pentagastrin challenge.

MANAGING SYMPTOMS OF THE CARCINOID SYNDROME

Several simple manoeuvres are available to reduce the symptoms of the carcinoid syndrome and include avoiding any food which has been found to precipitate attacks. Heart failure can be helped by diuretics, and bronchodilators may ease bronchospasm. Standard suppressants of gastrointestinal motility (e.g. loperamide) may reduce diarrhoea.

There are a few drugs such as parachlorophenylalanine, alpha-methyldopa and phenoxybenzamine which can provide relief from flushing or diarrhoea, but they all tend to have a short duration of activity before patients become refractory. Serotonin antagonists including ketanserin, cyproheptadine and methysergide may all benefit patients with diarrhoea but have little effect on flushing. Cyproheptadine is perhaps most often used and is usually started at a dose of 0.4 mg/kg/day in divided doses and then reduced to a level which produces the least side-effects. Ketanserin is reported to be better in controlling flushing episodes.

The advent of somatostatin analogues which seem to work by preventing the production of serotonin by a direct action on tumour cells, has significantly improved the symptomatic management of patients with the carcinoid syndrome. Octreotide may be given subcutaneously every 6 to 12 hours and produces useful palliation of all symptoms in over 50% of patients. It may be necessary to increase the dose from the usual starting level of 100 mg three times a day in order to get any response. Interestingly, anti-tumour effects of octreotide have also been reported, with tumour shrinkage being seen in up to 10% of patients.

Several studies have reported the value of interferon and objective tumour response has been reported in up to 20% of patients. More patients (up to 75%) will report improvement in diarrhoea, flushing or other symptoms, and urinary 5-HIAA excretion falls in up to 40%. In some centres, alpha-interferon may be accompanied by chemotherapy or hepatic artery embolization, although there is no clear evidence that such combined approaches are better than interferon alone.

Several new approaches for the treatment of carcinoid tumours are being investigated and one of the most promising is the use of ^{131}I-MIBG. Patients selected for this therapy should be those who have demonstrated uptake of the isotope during a diagnostic scan.

KEY POINTS

- Bronchial carcinoid tumours are uncommon.
- They are usually found as an incidental abnormality on Chest X-ray but may cause the symptoms of bronchial obstruction or the carcinoid syndrome.
- Surgery is the treatment of choice and is usually curative.
- The carcinoid syndrome can occur and is best managed symptomatically or with octreotide.

FURTHER READING

Norton J.A., Levin B., Jensen R.T. (1993) Carcinoid Tumors. In *Cancer: Principles and Practice of Oncology.* 4th edn. Edited by De Vita, Hellman and Rosenberg. Philadelphia: J.B. Lippincott and Co.

14 MALIGNANT MESOTHELIOMA

Malignant mesothelioma is the commonest primary pleural tumour. It is often a difficult tumour to diagnose, is seldom, if ever cured and usually causes the patients unpleasant symptoms that are hard to palliate. It is a tumour of mesothelial cells and can also, though less commonly, arise in the peritoneum.

ASBESTOS

It has been known for 30 years that malignant mesothelioma is usually associated with exposure to asbestos, although in 10% of cases there may be no clear history of occupational or environmental exposure. It is very important to take a careful occupational history as this may affect the patient's ability to obtain compensation. Asbestos was widely used in a number of industrial and manufacturing processes and as a building material and adequate controls over its use were not in place in the United Kingdom until the 1970s. The occupations most often associated with asbestos exposure and mesothelioma are listed in Table 14.1. There may be a very long interval, up to fifty years, between the known exposure and the development of the tumour.

Asbestos has different crystalline forms but it appears that amphiboles with linear fibres, particularly crocidolite (or 'blue' asbestos), cause mesothelioma.

Table 14.1   Occupations associated with a significant risk of exposure to asbestos

Asbestos mining and processing
Shipyard workers
Boilermakers
Power station builders
Central heating and ventilation engineers
Refrigeration engineers
Builders
Railway coach builders
Demolition workers
Joiners

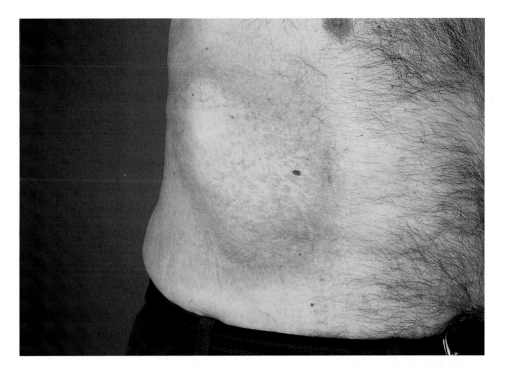

Plate 14.1 Photograph of the same patient as Plates 3.3 and 3.4 showing a mass growing through the chest wall. Pigmentation of the skin is due to radiotherapy.

A 68-year-old man, who worked as a plumber's fitter in the shipyards for many years, presented with increasing breathlessness and right-sided chest ache. There were dullness and reduced breath sounds throughout the right hemithorax and a firm swelling on the right chest wall (Plate 14.1). The chest X-ray (Plate 3.3) showed pleural calcification and thickening and appearances on the right side suggestive of a mesothelioma.

CT scanning (Plate 3.4) demonstrated the typical appearance of a mesothelioma and needle biopsy of the chest wall mass confirmed the presence of mesothelioma.

The patient received palliative radiotherapy to the right hemithorax, which improved the pain temporarily, but the tumour continued to grow. He became progressively more breathless and needed increasing doses of opiates. He died nine months after presentation.

Mesothelioma has also been reported in relatives of asbestos workers who may have been exposed to fibres by laundering working clothes and also in people who lived near asbestos manufacturing plants as children and were exposed to the dust.

There are currently over 700 deaths per year from mesothelioma in the United Kingdom and the incidence will probably continue to rise well into the next century because of the increasing use of asbestos without protection until 1970.

PATHOLOGY (see also Chapter 4)

The asbestos fibres are inhaled and, being sharp and straight, penetrate directly through the lung to the visceral pleura. The actual mechanism whereby these fibres induce malignant change remains unclear.

When the pleural tumour develops it is often associated with a pleural effusion. As the malignant process advances, the lung is gradually encased in a thick rim of tumour and there may be direct tumour extension into the chest wall, pericardium, contra-lateral pleura and, more rarely, through the diaphragm into the abdominal cavity.

Systemic metastases are more frequent than was once thought and the incidence of metastases at post mortem ranges from 30 to 80% in different series. However they seem to occur late in the course of the illness and are not often symptomatic. It is usually the local effects of the tumour that eventually cause death. The commonest sites of metastasis are lymph nodes, lung and liver, while bone and brain metastases are less common.

CLINICAL FEATURES

This tumour most commonly occurs in middle-aged or elderly men with an occupational history of asbestos exposure. The early symptoms are often minor and slowly progressive; this often results in the patients presenting late. The median time from first symptom to presentation is around six months.

The two commonest presenting symptoms are chest pain and dyspnoea. The chest pain usually starts as a vague ache on the affected side which gradually becomes more severe but is often rather diffuse and poorly localized and uncommonly associated with local tenderness. The increasing breathlessness is usually due to a pleural effusion rather than pulmonary constriction, at least in the early stages. Other common symptoms are cough, tiredness, anorexia and weight loss.

The commonest clinical finding at presentation is a pleural effusion and, as the tumour progresses, there is often evidence of marked loss of lung volume on the affected side. Sometimes (especially if thoracoscopy or repeated inter-costal tube drainage has been undertaken) small nodules or a larger mass may be felt in the chest wall (Plate 14.1).

INVESTIGATIONS

Radiology

The chest X-ray typically shows basal homogeneous opacification on one side due to pleural fluid and sometimes there is evidence of pleural thickening extending upwards around the lung edge. With more advanced disease, lobulated pleural shadowing may appear and, as the tumour progresses and encases the lung, there may be gradual loss of volume on the affected side. Calcified pleural plaques may be present, indicating previous asbestos exposure (Plate 3.3).

CT scanning is very useful in evaluating a patient with suspected mesothelioma. The appearances may be very characteristic, with an extensive area of pleural tumour encasing the lung (Plate 3.4) and often with an associated pleural effusion.

Although the chest X-ray and CT appearances can strongly suggest the diagnosis of mesothelioma, it is important to attempt to confirm the diagnosis histologically.

Pleural aspiration and biopsy

A patient suspected of having mesothelioma will usually have a significant pleural effusion at presentation. The first investigation after a chest X-ray should therefore be pleural aspiration. Pleural aspiration is performed simply under local anaesthesia. If there is doubt about the size or location of the pleural fluid, a brief ultrasound examination of the chest may help localize the best site for aspiration.

The fluid obtained is typically a blood-stained exudate. Unfortunately, cytological examination confirms the diagnosis in fewer than 50% of cases. This is partly because it can be difficult to distinguish between reactive mesothelial cells and malignant cells and, even if malignant cells are seen, it may be difficult to decide whether they come from a primary or secondary pleural tumour.

If pleural aspiration does not give the diagnosis, pleural biopsy, using an Abraham's needle, should be carried out. The diagnostic yield is probably no greater than 60% but it may give a more positive diagnosis than cytology. Cutting-needle or incisional biopsy of a pleural mass identified on CT scan or of a palpable chest-wall tumour gives the best chance of a definite diagnosis.

Following pleural aspiration or biopsy up to a third of patients will develop tumour seeding down the needle track. Radiotherapy may be helpful in preventing this problem (see below).

Thoracoscopy

If a clear diagnosis is not obtained by pleural aspiration and biopsy, thoracoscopy should be considered. With the advent of flexible, fibre-optic thoracoscopes, it is possible to carry this out under sedation and local anaesthesia, rather than putting the patient through a general anaesthetic. It may be possible to biopsy pleural nodules and masses under direct vision. Patients should not be subjected to thoracotomy unless there is a real possibility of a successful resection (see below).

Any patient with a persistent, undiagnosed pleural effusion, particularly if there is a history of asbestos exposure, should have a thoracoscopy to establish the diagnosis. This may be the only way of increasing the number of patients diagnosed early in the course of their illness.

MANAGEMENT

Malignant mesothelioma is a depressingly difficult tumour to treat. Because of the usual delays in presentation and diagnosis it is very unusual for any potentially curative procedure to be possible. Management is therefore primarily aimed at palliation and symptom control.

Surgery

Surgery has a very limited role because the patients usually present late, by which time there is often widespread pleural involvement. Very few patients can therefore be considered for surgical intervention.

There are two possible procedures. The first is a combined pneumonectomy and pleuro-pericardectomy. This is a major operation which is only possible in a fit patient with good respiratory reserve and cardiac function and a tumour that has not invaded significantly beyond the parietal pleura. It is sometimes necessary to resect the diaphragm and replace it with a dacron mesh.

Clearly, these limitations mean that the patients are highly selected and so, even in areas where the tumour is relatively frequent, experience of the procedure will be quite limited. It is therefore hard to assess its true value, particularly as it is associated with significant morbidity.

The second procedure is pleural stripping. Again the patients who are suitable for this treatment are those with limited disease and no significant parietal pleural involvement, and it is therefore probably only appropriate for those who present with recurrent pleural effusion rather than chest wall pain. It is a less morbid procedure and its advocates claim that it is an effective way of controlling the problem of effusion but it is not clear whether it also confers any survival benefit.

Radiotherapy

It is widely believed that mesothelioma is not at all responsive to radiotherapy. This is not entirely true. Certainly, as with most sarcomas, a high dose is probably needed to achieve any durable tumour control, but useful responses can be seen even with relatively low, palliative doses.

The typical late presentation and pattern of spread over the pleural surface means that high dose, radical radiotherapy is technically difficult, because the volume has to be very large and may include substantial amounts of normal tissues such as lung, heart and liver, that cannot tolerate the high dose needed. Techniques using combinations of megavoltage X-rays and electron fields have been described, but they are inevitably complex and it is not clear whether they are actually effective. Certainly there may be patients with a small volume of disease for whom radical radiotherapy might be an option but, as with surgery, until techniques for early diagnosis improve they will remain extremely uncommon.

Radiotherapy does have a limited but useful role in the palliation of patients with mesothelioma. Wide-field radiotherapy including the whole hemithorax from midline to lateral chest wall can be given to a dose of 30 Gy in ten fractions and provide reasonable, if short-lived, improvement in pain. It is necessary to treat a wide field because of the characteristic spread of the tumour and the poorly localized, diffuse nature of the pain.

This treatment is usually well tolerated. Nausea and vomiting may occur, especially if the diaphragm is included in the field and a significant amount of liver or stomach is irradiated. Treating a large volume of the lung to this dose is not really a problem even though it is higher than lung tolerance, because few patients survive long enough to get pneumonitis and anyway, if the tumour is widespread, the lung is effectively splinted and non-functional.

Palliative radiotherapy can also be useful in treating patients with troublesome masses growing through the chest wall especially down the tracks of biopsy needles and chest drains. These lumps can be painful, can fungate and bleed, or when large enough can be physically awkward for the patient. Usually a direct field to cover the mass can be used, but sometimes a pair of opposed glancing fields may be needed for a very large mass. A small area in an unfit patient could be adequately treated with a single fraction of 10–15 Gy, but higher doses such as 30 Gy in 10 fractions or 40 Gy in 15 fractions may be more appropriate if a large volume is treated or a more durable response is needed in a fitter patient.

Radiotherapy can also be used to prevent tumour seeding down the needle tracks. This occurs in about a third of patients who have had needle biopsies or repeated pleural drainage and for some it can be unpleasant and troublesome. A dose of 21 Gy in three daily fractions using orthovoltage X-rays or electrons and covering the area of the needle track or biopsy site may reduce the incidence of this problem.

Chemotherapy

Mesothelioma is not a chemotherapy-responsive tumour. A large number of drugs have been tried as single agents or in combination without any very encouraging results.

The most active agents are probably doxorubicin and carboplatin which both give objective responses rates of about 20%. We do not feel, however, that the activity of the drugs is high enough to recommend their routine use either for palliation or as an adjuvant after surgery.

Symptom control

Because so little can be achieved by surgery, chemotherapy or radiotherapy, it is very important that the patient's symptoms are controlled as well as possible. The major problems are recurrent pleural effusion and chest pain due to chest wall invasion. The management of these conditions is described in Chapter 10.

PROGNOSIS

The effect of any treatment on survival is uncertain as there have been no major controlled clinical trials. The median survival from diagnosis is 12 to 18 months, but a third of patients survive less than six months from the onset of their symptoms.

COMPENSATION

In the United Kingdom, the Medical Boarding Centre (Respiratory Diseases) evaluates claims in relation to possible asbestos-related lung disease. This includes mesothelioma and the Medical Boarding Centre can award compensation if, on the balance of probabilities, a mesothelioma is felt to be present, even in the absence of a definite histological diagnosis. Similar arrangements are present in many other industrialized countries. Alternatively, patients may take out a legal action against their previous employers on the basis that they failed to provide adequate protection from exposure to asbestos. Such actions may be successful irrespective of a successful application to the Medical Boarding Centre.

KEY POINTS

- Malignant mesothelioma is the commonest primary pleural tumour.
- It is strongly associated with exposure to asbestos dust, although the interval between exposure and the development of the tumour may be many years.
- The most frequent symptoms are chest wall pain and increasing breathlessness.
- The most frequent chest X-ray findings are pleural effusion and thickening.
- Establishing the histological diagnosis by pleural aspiration and biopsy may be difficult.
- Surgery is only possible for occasional patients who have very localized disease at presentation.
- Radiotherapy has a role in the palliation of chest wall pain and symptomatic masses and may prevent tumour seeding after pleural biopsy or thoracoscopy.

FURTHER READING

Butchart E.G., Wilkins M.F., Adams M., Antman K.H., Aisner J. (1989) Malignant Mesothelioma. In *Thoracic Oncology*. Edited by Roth J.A., Ruckdeschel J.C. and Weisenburger T.H. Philadelphia: W.B. Saunders Company.

INDEX